American Public Health Association
VITAL AND HEALTH STATISTICS MONOGRAPHS

Syphilis and Other Venereal Diseases

Syphilis and Other Venereal Diseases

WILLIAM J. BROWN / JAMES F. DONOHUE /
NORMAN W. AXNICK / JOSEPH H. BLOUNT /
NEAL H. EWEN / OSCAR G. JONES

HARVARD UNIVERSITY PRESS

Cambridge, Massachusetts, and London, England

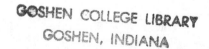

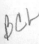

Library of Congress Catalog Card Number 77-88803
ISBN 0-674-86122-1
Printed in the United States of America

Preface

This monograph on syphilis and the other venereal diseases, sponsored by the American Public Health Association, is one of a series concerning vital and health statistics in the United States. Although syphilis mortality statistics are tabulated in greater detail for the three years 1959-1961 linked to the 1960 census data, much of the text is concerned with long-term trend data for morbidity, mortality, and epidemiologic activity related to the nationwide venereal disease control efforts which were initiated some years ago.

This report presents analyses of recent vital and health statistics, pertinent findings from special morbidity surveys and clinical studies, and discussions of trends. Its purpose is to review the history of the venereal diseases to reflect the important advances that have been made in the understanding of venereal diseases and methods of their prevention, control, and cure.

It was felt that a broad overall survey of these data would furnish a framework for understanding the advances made in venereal disease control, especially in the control of syphilis, and for evaluating the factors affecting further reductions in venereal disease incidence, prevalence, and debilitating late manifestations. Because only a broad survey of the data was made in this monograph, information regarding the qualification of the data and various aspects of the control program has been provided to give the interested reader a background for making additional interpretations of the data.

It is expected that this information will be useful to health officers, venereal disease control officers, social scientists, schools of medicine and public health, life and health insurance organizations, medical care program workers, research workers, students, and practicing physicians.

Contents

Tables

Figures

Foreword

Rapid advances in medical and allied sciences, changing patterns in medical care and public health programs, an increasingly health-conscious public, and the rising concern of voluntary agencies and government at all levels in meeting the health needs of the people necessitate constant evaluation of the country's health status. Such an evaluation, which is required not only for an appraisal of the current situation, but also to refine present goals and to gauge our progress toward them, depends largely upon a study of vital and health statistics records.

Opportunity to study mortality in depth emerges when a national census furnishes the requisite population data for the computation of death rates in demographic and geographic detail. Prior to the 1960 census of population there had been no comprehensive analysis of this kind. It seemed appropriate, therefore, to develop for intensive study a substantial body of death statistics for a three-year period centered around that census year.

A detailed examination of the country's health status must go beyond an examination of mortality statistics. Many conditions such as arthritis, rheumatism, and mental diseases are much more important as causes of morbidity than of mortality. Also, an examination of health status should not be based solely upon current findings, but should take into account trends and whatever pertinent evidence has been assembled through local surveys and from clinical experience.

The proposal for such an evaluation, to consist of a series of monographs, was made to the Statistics Section of the American Public Health Association in October 1958, and a Committee on Vital and Health Statistics Monographs was authorized. The members of this Committee and of the Editorial Advisory Subcommittee created later are:

Committee on Vital and Health Statistics Monographs

Mortimer Spiegelman, Chairman
Paul M. Densen, D. Sc.
Robert D. Grove, Ph.D.
Clyde V. Kiser, Ph.D.
Felix Moore
George Rosen, M.D., Ph.D.

William H. Stewart, M.D. (withdrew June 1964)
Conrad Taeuber, Ph.D.
Paul Webbink
Donald Young, Ph.D.

Editorial Advisory Subcommittee

Mortimer Spiegelman, Chairman
Duncan Clark, M.D.
E. Gurney Clark, M.D.
Jack Elinson, Ph.D.

Eliot Freidson, Ph.D. (withdrew
   February 1964)
Brian MacMahon, M.D., Ph.D.
Colin White, Ph.D.

The early history of this undertaking is described in a paper that was presented at the 1962 Annual Conference of the Milbank Memorial Fund.[1] The Committee on Vital and Health Statistics Monographs selected the topics to be included in the series and also suggested candidates for authorship. The frame of reference was extended by the Committee to include other topics in vital and health statistics than mortality and morbidity, namely fertility, marriage, and divorce. Conferences were held with authors to establish general guidelines for the preparation of the manuscripts.

Support for this undertaking in its preliminary stages was received from the Rockefeller Foundation, the Milbank Memorial Fund, and the Health Information Foundation. Major support for the required tabulations, for writing and editorial work, and for the related research of the monograph authors was provided by the United States Public Health Service (Research Grant CH 00075, formerly GM 08262). Acknowledgement should also be made to the Metropolitan Life Insurance Company for the facilities and time that were made available to Mr. Spiegelman, now retired from its service, who proposed and administered the undertaking and served as general editor. The National Center for Health Statistics, under the supervision of Dr. Grove and Miss Alice M. Hetzel, undertook the sizable tasks of planning and carrying out the extensive mortality tabulations for the period 1959-1961. Dr. Taeuber arranged for the cooperation of the Bureau of the Census at all stages of the project in many ways, principally by furnishing the required population data used in computing death rates and by undertaking a large number of varied special tabulations. As the sponsor of the project, the American Public Health Association furnished assistance through Dr. Thomas R. Hood, its Deputy Executive Director.

[1]Mortimer Spiegelman, "The Organization of the Vital and Health Statistics Monograph Program," *Emerging Techniques in Population Research (Proceedings of the 1962 Annual Conference of the Milbank Memorial Fund;* New York: Milbank Memorial Fund, 1963), p. 230. See also Mortimer Spiegelman, "The Demographic Viewpoint in the Vital and Health Statistics Monographs Project of the American Public Health Association," *Demography,* vol. 3, No. 2 (1966), p. 574.

Because of the great variety of topics selected for monograph treatment, authors were given an essentially free hand to develop their manuscripts as they desired. Accordingly, the authors of the individual monographs bear the full responsibility for their manuscripts, and their opinions and statements do not necessarily represent the viewpoints of the American Public Health Association or of the agencies with which they are affiliated.

Berwyn F. Mattison, M.D.
Executive Director
American Public Health Association

Notes on Tables

1. Regarding 1959-61 mortality data:
   a. Deaths relate to those occurring in the United States (including Alaska and Hawaii);
   b. Deaths are classified by place of residence (if pertinent);
   c. Fetal deaths are excluded;
   d. Deaths of unknown age, marital status, nativity, or other characteristics have not been distributed into the known categories, but are included in their totals;
   e. Deaths were classified by cause according to the *Seventh Revision of the International Statistical Classification of Diseases, Injuries, and Causes of Death* (Geneva: World Health Organization, 1957);
   f. All death rates are average annual rates per 100,000 population in the category specified, as recorded in the United States census of April 1, 1960;
   g. Age-adjusted rates were computed by the direct method using the age distribution of the total United States population in the census of April 1, 1940 as a standard.[1]
2. Symbols used in tables of data:
   ---Data not available;
   ...Category not applicable;
   -Quantity zero;
   0.0 Quantity more than zero but less than 0.05;
   *Figure does not meet the standard of reliability of precision:
   a) Rate or ratio based on less than 20 deaths;
   b) Percentage or median based on less than 100 deaths;
   c) Age-adjusted rate computed from age-specific rates where more than half of the rates were based on frequencies of less than 20 deaths.
3. Geographic classification:[2]
   a. Standard Metropolitan Statistical Areas (SMSA's): except in the New England States, "an SMSA is a county or a group of contiguous counties which contains at least one city of 50,000 inhabitants or more or 'twin cities' with a combined population of at least 50,000 in the 1960 census. In addition, contiguous counties are included in an SMSA if, according to specified criteria, they are (a) essentially metropolitan in character and (b) socially and economically integrated with the central city or cities." In New England, the Division of Vital Statistics of the National Center for Health Statistics uses, instead of the definition just cited, Metropolitan State Economic Areas (MSEA's) established by the Bureau of the Census, which are made up of county units.

[1]Mortimer Spiegelman and H.H. Marks, "Empirical Testing of Standards for the Age Adjustment of Death Rates by the Direct Method," *Human Biology*, 38:280 (September 1966).

[2]National Center for Health Statistics, *Vital Statistics of the United States, 1960*, vol. II, *Mortality*, Part A, sec. 7, p. 8.

b. Metropolitan and nonmetropolitan: "Counties which are included in SMSA's or, in New England, MSEA's are called metropolitan counties; all other counties are classified as nonmetropolitan."

c. Metropolitan counties may be separated into those containing at least one central city of 50,000 inhabitants or more or twin cities as specified previously, and into metropolitan counties without a central city.

4. Sources:

In addition to any sources specified in the figures, text tables, and appendix tables, the deaths and death rates for the period 1959-61 are derived from special tabulations made at the National Center for Health Statistics, Public Health Service, U.S. Department of Health, Education, and Welfare, for the American Public Health Association.

Syphilis and Other Venereal Diseases

1 / The History of Syphilis

Probably no other disease, communicable or chronic, has been as widely studied as syphilis. Papers and articles, enough to fill many large volumes, have been written on the subject. From its recognized appearance in Europe over four centuries ago to the present time, syphilis has caused great concern and controversy. Control has always been difficult; eradication, to this point in time, impossible. Despite all the efforts made to combat the disease, syphilis continues to be a major health problem in most countries today.

The attitudes toward syphilis held by both scientists and laymen are often less than objective. Most communicable diseases are studied empirically to determine cause, mode of transmission, treatment, and methods of prevention. Efforts are usually made to treat existing infection, inhibit spread, and disseminate information on preventive measures. Syphilis, however, has been shrouded in secrecy, clothed in superstition and ignorance, and viewed more as a character weakness than a communicable disease. Such attitudes are still held and are no more effective in eradicating the disease today than they have been in the past.

Much discussion and debate has centered around the controversial geographic origin of the disease. Two opposing schools of thought have developed on this subject, each trying to outpublish the other to prove its point. Students of the pre-Columbian school contend that syphilis is a disease as old as man himself and has been present in all civilizations from earliest times. Proponents of the Columbian school claim syphilis to be a disease of the Western hemisphere which was not present in Europe until introduced there by the sailors of Columbus. Each argument has certain points in its favor, but absolute proof of one or total refutation of the other is impossible. However, the ingenuity and persistence displayed by each side in attempting to prove its theory is commendable, and in retrospect rather fascinating.

PRE-COLUMBIAN SCHOOL

The pre-Columbian school maintains simply that syphilis has plagued mankind from the days of his earliest recorded history, as evidenced by literary and historical sources.[1] The Bible is frequently cited as a reference, for it contains several passages which can conceivably be interpreted as pertaining to syphilis: Job 2:7: "So went Satan forth from the presence of the Lord, and smote Job with sore boils from the sole of his foot unto his crown;" Job 19:20: "My bone cleaveth to my skin and to my flesh, and I am escaped with the skin of my teeth." And David in Psalms 38:5,7 says, "My wounds stink and are corrupt because of my foolishness. . . For my loins are filled with a loathesome disease; and there is no soundness in my flesh."

Other passages from the Bible are more specific. In Exodus 20:5 the Second Commandment says in part: "for I the Lord thy God am a jealous God, visiting the iniquity of the fathers upon the children unto the third and fourth generation of them that hate me. . ." Although today we know that inherited (congenital) syphilis is transmissible only to the second generation, this passage is significant because syphilis is one of the few known communicable diseases that can be passed from one generation to another.

In Jeremiah 31:29-30 we find another reference to what might be congenital syphilis: "In those days they shall say no more; The fathers have eaten a sour grape, and the children's teeth are set on edge. But everyone shall die from his own iniquity; every man that eateth the sour grape, his teeth shall be set on edge." This could be a description of Hutchinson's teeth, a condition resulting from congenital syphilis, in which teeth are imperfectly formed with notched edges, incomplete cusps, and irregular spacing.

And still again in Numbers 12:12: "Let her not be as one dead, of whom the flesh is half consumed when he cometh out of his mother's womb." This is suggestive of a macerated syphilitic still-born.

Deuteronomy 28:27-29 could be a description of syphilis stages: "The Lord will smite thee with the botch of Egypt, and with the emerods, and with the scab, and the itch, whereof thou canst not be healed. The Lord shall smite thee with madness, and blindness, and astonishment of heart: And thou shall grope at noonday, as the blind gropeth in darkness, and thou shalt not prosper in thy ways: and thou shalt be only oppressed and spoiled ever more, and no man shall save thee."

Essentially no biblical passage can be cited as indisputable evidence of the antiquity of syphilis. Clinical detail is lacking; concern with the poetic presentation of ideas is more prominent than the specifics of history and medicine. Though these passages cannot be considered winning arguments for the pre-Columbian school, they do present literary evidence of the possibility of syphilis being an age-old scourge of man.

Outside of the Bible, there are few literary references to conditions which could be of syphilitic origin. Hippocrates in 460 B.C. described genital lesions which followed sexual exposure. During the first century A.D., the Roman physician Celsus described hard and soft genital sores. The treatment of nontraumatic aneurysm of the aorta was mentioned by Greek and other writers hundreds of years before the time of Columbus. The word *buba* was in use at the time of the discovery of America and meant a scab, a wound, or a little tumor of matter. When syphilis was recognized as a disease with multiple visible lesions, the plural form *bubas* was given to these lesions. *Bubas* came to be employed in Spain in the singular sense as the name for syphilis. However, literature written between the fall of the Roman Empire and Columbus's discovery of America contains little helpful information.

Critics of the pre-Columbian theory state that syphilis has been accurately named "The Great Imitator" and that the ailments described in ancient texts are vague and could as easily refer to other diseases—pityriasis rosea, urticaria pigmentosa, psoriasis, chicken pox, leprosy, scabies, and yaws—as to syphilis. They also observe that none of the accounts relate the cutaneous lesions of secondary syphilis to primary symptoms, nor are symptoms of early syphilis connected with the disorders of late stages.

As for the claims of syphilitic genital symptoms during the pre-Columbian era, the critics contend that a description of a typical Hunterian chancre is notably missing in the ancient writings and that chancroidal ulcerations and phagedenic sores are not, of course, syphilitic. With reference to the claims of aneurysm in ancient times in the Old World, those in favor of the Columbian theory feel it sufficient to point out that not all aneurysms of the aorta are syphilitic. Those of the Columbian school also point out that bones in the Old World showing gummatous changes may be attributed to arthritis deformans. They contend that there is a confusion of syphilis with yaws in some of the languages and that "bubas" is often the term applied to yaws even now in some South American countries.

Whatever the answer, it is impossible to determine the origin of syphilis by compiling a literary sampler. Consequently the advocates of the pre-Columbian school turn also to the field of historical events for support.

Certain historical events during the Middle Ages and Renaissance are used to support the theory of the European origin of syphilis. There is general agreement that during the very late fifteenth and early sixteenth centuries syphilis epidemics swept Europe with unprecedented intensity and virulence. So severe were these epidemics that thousands of people are believed to have died, primarily or exclusively because of the pathogenicity of the syphilis organism during the secondary stage. To cope with the problem, authorities banished infected persons from towns, often on pain of death. When consulted for advice, doctors and astrologers responded by devising countless potions and devices which usually benefited them more than their patients. Finally the pandemic quality of the disease lessened. Sometime in the sixteenth century, syphilis either lost its virulence or its host (man) became more resistant; while infections still occurred, epidemics accompanied by rapid death disappeared. Thus has the state of the disease remained to the present day.

The factors contributing to these epidemics are probably multiple and certainly obscure. Devotees of the pre-Columbian origin of syphilis in the Old World point to specific historical events which may have influenced the spread of infection. The preceding four centuries saw seven major crusades and thousands of pilgrimages to the eastern Mediterranean area. Epidemics also occurred during the Renaissance, an era of increased travel and trade between nations and peoples who previously had been relatively isolated. If, in fact, different peoples had infectious diseases peculiar to themselves—travel, trade, and pilgrimages could certainly have been factors in outbreaks of syphilis and other diseases.

This explanation, however, does not account for the severity of the epidemics which occurred. There had always been some communication between Europe and Asia Minor. Some writers have suggested that a pathogenic mutation of the treponeme occurred within the European population itself, or that a virulent strain was introduced from America into a population previously afflicted with another form of treponematosis. Both of these are possibilities but they cannot be proven.

Still other considerations are involved. Papal bulls in 1490 and 1505 abolished leper houses, allowing thousands of people to wander about Europe, carrying with them leprosy and many other diseases. Holcomb, quoting Matthew of Paris, says that shortly before their abolition leper houses numbered around 19,000.[2] It is possible that the "freeing" of lepers, many of whom may well have been syphilitic, accounts in part for the epidemics. But, again, this does not explain the severity of the epidemics or take into account the fact that many of the freed lepers, even if infected with syphilis, would have progressed to noninfectious latent stages by the time of their release. Singly or together, these factors do not conclusively establish the presence of syphilis in Europe prior to Columbus's voyage to America.

COLUMBIAN SCHOOL

Evidence suggesting that syphilis was a disease native to America is almost entirely circumstantial.[3] Those espousing the Columbian theory claim that syphilis was acquired from the Indians and carried to Europe by Columbus on his return to Spain. There is disagreement concerning the dates, places of appearance, and routes by which the disease traveled, but it is generally agreed that syphilis was present throughout Europe by 1500. Its rapid spread and virulence are offered as evidence that syphilis was a new infection to which Europeans had no resistance. The journals of physicians indicate that they were baffled by and unable to cope with this new disease.

Pusey[4] searched the ancient texts to trace the origin of syphilis in Europe to Columbus's mariners. The historical facts seem to be made to order to explain how Columbus's small crew could have started the conflagration of syphilis that spread across Europe.

One might suppose that Columbus's crew and his Indians had syphilis and spread it. Some of the infected Spaniards, along with mercenaries from all parts of Europe, joined the army of Charles VIII, the French King. In 1494 Charles VIII and his army crossed the Alps into Italy for the conquest of Naples. (However, there is no proof that any of Columbus's crew actually joined Charles's army.)

In the spring of 1495 a violent plague, which most contemporary records attribute to syphilis, broke out among Charles's troops, forcing a disorganized retreat and breaking up the army. Soldiers made their way home as best they could, spreading syphilis as they went. Most contemporary records attribute the beginning of the epidemic in Europe to the dispersal of the mercenaries of Charles VIII's army over Europe. However, some historians feel that the epidemiology of syphilis as known today makes it incredible that the small group of mariners that accompanied Columbus could have launched such an epidemic.

Opponents argue that if the disease was introduced by Columbus and his sailors, it would have been mentioned in the otherwise detailed chronicles of the voyage.

Columbus noted in his journal that there was no sickness on his ship, excepting that of an old man who was troubled with gravel. Some feel that the journal kept by Columbus for the information of Ferdinand and Isabella was prepared to show his expedition in the most glowing colors, particularly in view of the trouble he had getting backing for the expedition. An example of this is given by Harrison who notes that "Columbus said that the first voyage took 33 days, whereas it took 71 days."[5]

Dr. Diza de Isla was practicing in Barcelona when Columbus's first expedition returned in 1493. He wrote that syphilis was unknown prior to 1493 and that it was introduced into Barcelona by the men of Columbus's vessels on their return from Española. He stated that he treated some members of Columbus's crew who were infected with "bubas" or "the serpentine disease," later called syphilis.

As syphilis spread, each nation blamed the disease on enemies or rivals. Italians called it the Spanish or French disease; the French called it the Italian disease; the English called it the French disease. Spaniards called it the Disease of Española (Haiti). For centuries syphilis was generally referred to as the *morbus gallicus,* the French disease.

Proponents of the Old World origin of syphilis point out that the term *morbus gallicus* (or mal franzoso, mal français, the grosse verole) for skin diseases that may have been chiefly syphilitic had been used in parts of Europe for many years prior to the discovery of America. Some proponents of the New World origin of syphilis point out that this very multiplicity of names came into use about 1493 and in succeeding years and is an indication that syphilis was a disease previously unknown in the countries that named it after their neighbors. Syphilis acquired its present name when Hieronymi Fracastorius wrote a poem published in 1530 about a shepherd named Syphilus who was afflicted with a strange infection.

Other evidence supporting the New World origin of syphilis is based on examinations of bones, skulls, and mummies uncovered by archaeologists. Herbert Williams, in an extensive article on diseased bones, indicated that remains from graves in the Old World show no damage positively attributable to syphilis.[6] Other scholars disagree with him, contending that some specimens from European cities definitely show signs of syphilis deterioration.

Considering the arguments and counter-arguments which each side offers, it would seem unlikely that either the pre-Columbian or Columbian theory is wholly correct.

While yaws and perhaps other spirochetal diseases even more closely related to syphilis undoubtedly existed in other parts of the world, the disease syphilis, as we know it, probably first appeared in Europe in the fifteenth century; possibly by spontaneous mutation of a spirochete already present and possibly by introduction from without, perhaps from the Americas. With this in mind, many present day authors have moved to the middle of the road and suggested that certain elements in both theories may have validity. Thomas Cockburn[7] and E. H. Hudson[8, 9, 10] are leading contemporary spokesmen for what might be called the Evolutionary School on the origin of syphilis.

EVOLUTIONARY SCHOOL

Cockburn's Theory

Cockburn's evolutionary theory[11] is based on a hypothesis in which all parasites are descended from free-living organisms and the different races of man from a common ancestor. Some thousands or perhaps millions of years ago, a treponemal parasite attached itself to man (or man's ancestors) and since that time, a symbiotic evolution of both host and parasite has taken place. According to this theory, man probably originated in Africa or Central Asia and, during one or more of the four most recent glacial advances, migrated in small groups or tribes to different parts of the earth, carrying with him treponemal infection. After glaciers retreated, sea levels rose, leaving man isolated in several parts of the world until the relatively recent development of means of intercontinental travel. The thousands of years of isolation produced a degree of speciation among different groups of men and their respective treponemes. This resulted in the appearance of different racial and ethnic groups and the differentiation of the genus *Treponema* into the species *pallidum, pertenue,* and *carateum* – the etiologic agents of syphilis, yaws, and pinta, respectively. (For a description of yaws and pinta, see Chapter 9, "International Venereal Disease Control.")

Symbiotic evolution has produced situations today in which host and parasite are peculiarly adapted to one another and to the ecological conditions under which both survive. For example, pinta, despite numerous opportunities to spread elsewhere in the past four centuries, has remained confined to a small part of Central America because of the dependence of the parasite on the native host, the only host susceptible to infection. *T. pertenue,* the etiologic agent causing yaws, is less selective of host, but requires a humid, tropical climate, poor hygiene and health, and crowded living conditions in order to be transmitted cutaneously from one person to another. *T. pallidum,* the organism causing syphilis, is a delicate genitotrophic strain of treponeme which evolved in the cooler climates of Europe as better hygiene and higher standards of living developed.

One type of treponematosis cannot be introduced to an area where another type is indigenous. Venereal syphilis, therefore, can rarely be transmitted to persons in an endemic yaws area, because most persons have acquired yaws in childhood and are immune to the venereal transmission of another treponemal infection. Similarly, yaws cannot survive in Europe because of the cooler climate, the inhibiting effect of clothing, and better health and hygiene.

Cockburn presents two corollary theories which by inference could account for the occurrence of epidemics of syphilis and other communicable diseases in Europe during the late fifteenth and early sixteenth centuries. In a small, isolated population, pathogenic infections are low-grade, chronic, and nonfatal, for pathogenic epidemic infections would eliminate their host and thus disappear themselves. In larger, diversified populations such as those which developed in Europe under feudalism and the Renaissance, acute, fatal infections became a possibility and a not uncommon occurrence. They spread through a given group or area, killing some, but not liquidating the entire group. This characteristic of infectious diseases might be the cause of the sudden advent of syphilis epidemics in Europe in post-Columbian decades and an explanation of the dramatic recognition of the disease as such.

Cockburn completely discounts the theory that syphilis was suddenly introduced to Europe from America by Columbus and other explorers. Instead, he suggests that the exploration of the world and the emergence of syphilis are by-products of the Renaissance, which inspired man not only to travel but to improve his living standards and increase his knowledge. Venereal treponemal infections had developed in Europe in the decades or centuries prior to the Renaissance, but had been poorly understood and not always differentiated from other diseases with similar cutaneous manifestations. That it was recognized at the time Columbus voyaged to America was pure coincidence.

Hudson's Theory

A second evolutionary theory on the origin of treponemal infection has been advanced by Hudson as a unitarian concept of treponemal evolution.[12, 13, 14] He also sees man migrating about the globe from his ancestral home in Central Asia or Africa, but at this point suggests that treponemal infections have remained unchanged since man left his original home, and that treponemato*ses* is a misnomer for what should be treponemato*sis*. Clinical variations among treponemal infections are due to health, hygiene, mode of transmission, and geographic distribution rather than to etiological differences.

Yaws predominates in hot, humid areas where hygiene is poor and where cutaneous lesions can be transmitted by close physical contact in crowded sleeping and living quarters. Endemic syphilis (bejel) is found primarily in hot, dry areas such as Asia Minor and grassland Africa. In these regions, dry climatic conditions prevent generalized cutaneous lesions and transmission. Instead, manifestations appear on moist areas of the body, for example, in the mouth as mucuous patches, and in the ano-genital region. Transmission is by means of hands, mouth, or contaminated intermediate objects rather than casual physical contact. Where climatic zones are in transition, as in the Egyptian Sudan, both yaws and endemic syphilis are present.

The appearance of venereal syphilis is related not so much to climate (although it is primarily a temperate zone disease), but rather to hygiene and standards of living. As health and personal and environmental hygiene improved, the conditions permitting the non-sexual spread of treponemal infections disappeared, and venereal syphilis finally was recognized. In a sense the appearance of syphilis is an unwelcome by-product of man's increased knowledge and urbanization. Like Cockburn, Hudson views the recognition of syphilis at the time of the discovery of America as coincidental.

Hudson's concept, if valid, would explain why the lesions of treponemal infections are often clinically indistinguishable, why all four produce reactive serologic tests, and why under darkfield examination treponemes from all lesions are identical. But it cannot explain why venereal syphilis causes extensive damage in congenital infections and in central-nervous-system involvement, while yaws, pinta, and bejel do not.

In general it may be said that the distribution of treponemal disease is worldwide. The spectrum of distribution seems to narrow as one considers in order bejel (endemic syphilis), yaws, and pinta. The mode of transmission for venereal syphilis is largely through sexual contact. The mode of transmission for the others is largely nonvenereal. The above differences may be due partly to the social and physical environment in which the host finds himself: the more primitive the culture, the less venereal transmission. One might speculate that these environmental variations determine the differences in the early and possibly even the late manifestations of the disease in the individual.

Both Hudson and Cockburn place a great amount of reliance on our knowledge of the treponeme itself. However, we do not know the genetic structure or the method of reproduction of *T. pallidum,* nor are we able to culture the organism. For Hudson to state that the etiologic agents of treponemal infections are identical or for Cockburn to assign them to the same genus but different species raises many as yet unanswered questions. The evolutionary approach these authors have used appears somewhat more convincing than the literary-historical approach of earlier authors in unraveling the mystery of the origin of syphilis, but it is doubtful that anyone will satisfactorily resolve the controversy over the origin of syphilis.

2 / Evolution of Treatment

The earliest reported hygienic measures for disease control appear in Exodus, where Moses provides quarantine laws to prevent epidemics of different diseases. Persons suspected of having communicable diseases were banished from the camp and were not allowed to return until they appeared to be healthy. Often the outcasts included those who suffered from dermatological disorders; people with leprosy, yaws, scabies, and a variety of other diseases with cutaneous manifestations were considered leprous and were ostracized. The quarantine technique must have been particularly severe on persons suffering from chronic diseases or whose symptoms were permanent, for they were rarely welcomed back to the tribe. Quarantine measures of this kind, based only on clinical symptoms, are certainly not 100 percent effective, for many diseases can be infectious but asymptomatic. Yet despite their imperfections, the quarantine measures used by Moses were probably beneficial in promoting the public health, for, by isolating at least some of the infected, the chance of spreading disease to healthy persons was reduced. The quarantine system of dealing with diseases continued for centuries and is sometimes used even today.

While the use of quarantine indicates that man has long employed certain preventive measures for disease, there is little indication that he possessed adequate therapy for a given disease once it had been acquired. In those passages from the Bible allegedly dealing with syphilis, there is no indication of treatment. Hippocrates suggests no cure. The Romans had no effective treatment for genital lesions. Astrologers and charlatans had many suggestions, but their variety and abundance suggest that none of them were effective or respected for very long.

At the time of the syphilis epidemic in Europe, many treatments were attempted. The most common of these "cures" were compounds of mercury, a treatment which Arabs had used for centuries for scabies and yaws. In 1363 Guy de Chauliac wrote his *Grande Chirugie* in which mercury was prescribed for scabies. This text became well known in Europe, so that when syphilis later devastated the continent, its similarity to scabies suggested the use of mercury. Paracelsus is often credited with the introduction of mercury, but it is more likely that he merely popularized the idea.

Paracelsus also suggested arsenic as therapy around 1530, but this treatment was rarely used after its fatal toxic effects became known. For four hundred years, up to the time salvarsan was introduced, mercury was essentially the only therapy for syphilis, and, while not a cure, it was superior to any other treatment available. Its chief disadvantage however proved to be the disastrous side effects that developed when it was improperly administered. Mercury originally was given in four ways: orally, by inunction, by salves, and by fumigation. Treatment schedules varied from a specified time period in some courses to the disappearance of symptoms in others. Variation in schedules depended upon the technique of the physician and the affluence of the patient.

When inunction was used, mercury was rubbed several times daily on different parts of the body, the metal being absorbed cutaneously. Mercurial salve plasters used the same principle, except that the metal was kept in continuous close contact with the skin. Treatment by fumigation was probably the least effective and most arduous treatment method. A person was placed in a closed compartment, only the head protruding, while a fire was set under the cabinet, raising the temperature and vaporizing the mercury. Fumigation treatments were not long popular, probably because of the ordeal involved. Mercury from oral doses was absorbed internally.

The four processes were evaluated by the amount of salivation they produced in a patient. For, in theory, salivation was supposed to carry away venereal poison. Three pints of saliva daily was considered good prognosis. If a patient did not produce this amount the quantity of mercury was increased. It has been recorded that up to sixteen pounds of mercury was given in a single course of treatment.[1]

Although Stokes[2] has demonstrated that in very limited amounts in special situations, mercury therapy was of some slight value in treating syphilis, the side effects of sixteenth century mercurial treatment were severe. The amount given to patients was frequently excessive, causing severe ulcerations of the gums and palate, loosening of the teeth, gastrointestinal disorders, and deterioration of bones.

J. Johnston Abraham tells the story of one of the early victims of improperly administered mercury. His account runs as follows:

> The first sufferer to rebel in print against the treatment was Ulrich von Hutten, a German poet and a friend of the great

scholar Erasmus. He said he had had six treatments in eight years. Each day of his treatment he had one to four inunctions, he was kept in bed in one room at a high temperature, and he was heavily clothed to produce sweating. This went on for twenty to thirty days, during which he was not allowed out of his room. According to him, his jaws, tongue, lips, and palate became ulcerated, his gums swelled, his teeth loosened and fell out. Saliva dripped continuously from his mouth, and his breath became intolerably foetid. The whole apartment where he was being treated stank intolerably, and the cure was so hard to suffer he felt he would rather choose to die than to submit to it further. Yet in spite of all these treatments, he says he relapsed . . .3

Ulrich later tried guaiacum which he claims cured his infection. Abraham states that he died at the age of 35.

Though in its limited way mercury was the preferred treatment of the pre-arsphenamine era, it was certainly not the only one tried. A popular potion of the sixteenth century was a decoction of guaiacum wood administered orally. This West Indies wood was supposedly used as a syphilis cure by American Indians. When proven ineffective, the popularity of guaiacum diminished. Another drug, introduced by the Portuguese, was called "China Root." Imported from Goa, this substance soon proved ineffective. Sarsaparilla and sassafras preparations then had their vogue, with sarsaparilla remaining popular up until this century. It still has adherents who extol it as a health tonic.

None of the treatments were certain, and all were slow. Because results were not dramatic when mercury was administered in small amounts, many practitioners prescribed what often proved to be fatal doses. Short intensive treatments were considered most effective. As might be expected when no cure for a disease is known, charlatans cheated many patients with promises of quick, permanent cures. After collecting their fees, they disappeared before relapses and side effects from toxic dosages set in.

Dual infections of syphilis and gonorrhea caused confusion among physicians, many of whom thought that the symptoms were simply different stages of the same disease. Lacking today's diagnostic tools, physicians assumed that the discharge of gonorrhea, followed by primary and secondary symptoms of syphilis, was the chronological clinical sequence of syphilis. It was believed that the site of infection accounted for the difference in symptoms. When infection was acquired externally, a chancre appeared; when inoculation was internal (intra-urethral), a discharge was the first symptom.

Iodides were introduced to syphilis therapy in 1821 and were very popular in France during the nineteenth century. They were non-specific and valueless in primary or secondary stages and in treating pregnant women. Effectiveness was limited mainly to reducing granulomatous and cutaneous lesions of late syphilis. They could be administered either orally or intravenously, and, because their systemic effect was slight, large dosages could be used. As a conditioner prior to the administration of arsenicals, iodide therapy was helpful in preventing Herxheimer reactions in patients with active syphilis.

Bismuth, first introduced in 1884, did not gain wide acceptance as a therapeutic agent until after World War I. In the following years it almost completely displaced mercury as heavy metal therapy for syphilis. Its spirillicidal action was greater and toxic effects less than those of mercury. Intramuscular injection was preferred to oral administration. Bismuth was valuable in conjunction with the arsphenamines as it inhibited multiplication of spirochetes and could be tolerated by patients who reacted to arsenic.

Tellurium, vanadium, platinum, and gold were used experimentally in treatment but never became popular. They were less effective than mercury or bismuth.

In this century syphilis therapy has changed radically as a result of research discoveries. In 1905 Schaudinn and Hoffman demonstrated that *T. pallidum* was the etiologic organism causing syphilis, solving a problem that had baffled medicine for centuries. Donne had actually detected *T. pallidum* in 1837 and at that time suggested that it was the cause of infection, but he later withdrew his hypothesis. In 1906 Wassermann, Bruck, and Neisser revolutionized syphilis diagnosis when they produced a complement fixation test which detected infection from analysis of specimens of blood or spinal fluid. Later in the same year darkfield microscopy was introduced as a diagnostic tool. The year 1907 became a landmark in syphilology when Paul Ehrlich developed an arsenical treatment which he hoped would provide a cure for syphilis in a single injection. This, of course, was not the case. Although arsenicals were sometimes effective, cessation of treatment was usually followed by relapse. Nevertheless, arsenicals were to remain the treatment of choice for syphilis until penicillin was introduced.

For several years there was no standard arsenical therapy. Treatment schedules varied according to the practitioner and the reliability of the patient, and practically every major syphilologist in the country had his own preferred dosages. Eventually the Health Section of the League of Nations met and discussed the problem. United States participation in this meeting resulted in the formation of the Cooperative Clinical Group which, after analyzing the records of thousands of clinic cases, recommended a seventy-week schedule as standard treatment.[4]

Several different arsenicals were used as treatment, including arsphenamine, neoarsphenamine, sulfarsphenamine, oxophenarsine hydrochloride, and tryparsamide. Arsenical treatment was arduous and accompanied by complications. Poisoning from improperly supervised treatment or from individual hypersensitivity was not uncommon. Aplastic anemia, exfoliative dermatitis, hemorrhagic encephalitis, and purpura hemmorhagica were not infrequent and often resulted in death. These medical problems were further intensified by the difficulty of case-holding. Because of the painful injections and long-term nature of the treatment, many patients returned for subsequent therapy only occasionally or not at all. It is estimated that prior to penicillin perhaps only 20-25 percent of the patients who ever received treatment were actually treated adequately enough to arrest their infections.[5, 6]

After observing the beneficial effects of malarial fever on persons with psychoses, Wagner von Jauregg introduced fever therapy as treatment in 1917.[7] He discovered that *T. pallidum* could be destroyed or its reproduction and virulence inhibited by raising body temperatures. Fevers were induced by inoculating a patient with a fever-producing disease, such as malaria or typhoid, or by raising the temperature externally. Immediately obvious were the complications resulting from fevers created by inoculation with another disease, so other techniques were employed. The famous inventor and industrialist Charles Kettering became involved in the field of syphilis when he developed a "fever box" reminiscent of the fumigation treatment of the sixteenth century. With only his head protruding, the luckless recipient of this imaginative approach was placed in the box while body temperature was maintained at 106.7°F for a prescribed number of hours. During the process an attendant or nurse occasionally bathed the patient's brow with cool water. Careful temperature control had to be maintained, for a slight rise could have resulted in death by roasting. Arsenicals were thoughtfully administered in conjunction with the fever-box ordeal.

Even though artificial fevers were favored over those induced by malaria, and though some positive therapeutic gains were achieved by means of fever therapy (particularly in neurosyphilis), the treatment was hazardous, unpredictable, and generally unsatisfactory. Fever therapy disappeared with the advent of penicillin.

Immediately prior to and during World War II, a new, intensive arsenotherapy schedule was developed by Dr. Harry Eagle at Johns Hopkins University. This schedule was fairly effective and had the added advantage of being the shortest of the arsenical schedules, requiring only eight or ten weeks for completion. Eagle's treatment would probably have increased in popularity but for the discovery of penicillin.

In 1928 Alexander Fleming had observed the effect of penicillin on bacterial cultures, but it was not until 1943 that Dr. John Mahoney, working in a Public Health Service hospital on Staten Island, demonstrated the efficacy of the drug as therapy for syphilis.[8] Penicillin was first made available to the Public Health Service in June 1944, for use in rapid treatment centers. Administered at first in conjunction with arsenicals and bismuth, it soon became the only treatment for syphilis. The first penicillin used required intramuscular injections at two to three hour intervals around the clock and was practical only for inpatient care. The development of delayed absorption preparations soon made possible outpatient care with single daily shots on schedules of seven to ten days. In 1953 benzathine penicillin G, a repository form of penicillin, was developed, making possible the effective one-shot treatment of syphilis. Since that time 2.4 million units of this preparation has been the recommended treatment for early syphilis.

The decrease in the number of reported cases which began in 1949 caused federal grants to states to be sharply reduced or eliminated in 1954. Many public clinics were closed in the expectation that the eradication effort could be completed by private physicians. Unfortunately, the morbidity trends of the past decade indicate that syphilis remains a problem and that more than penicillin in the hands of private physicians is necessary to effect eradication.

3 / The Diagnosis and Treatment of Syphilis

The Causative Organism

The causative organism of syphilis is the *Treponema pallidum,* a spirilliform organism characterized by thinness, motility (slow forward and backward movement, rotation about the long axis, and a slight bending, twisting, or undulation from side to side), and the closeness and regularity of 6 to 14 corkscrew-like spirals. It is a delicate organism with tapering ends, about 6 to 15 microns in length (approximately the diameter of a normal red blood cell), and of uniform cylindrical thickness of approximately 0.25 micron. Although a number of mammalian species are readily infected by *Treponema pallidum,* man is its only natural host.

Outside of the host, the *Treponema pallidum* is extremely frail and is easily destroyed by a variety of physical and chemical agents. Such things as heat, drying, and soap and water will bring about its immediate destruction. Because *Treponema pallidum* cannot thrive outside the human body, syphilis is almost always contracted by the direct transference of the microorganisms from one person to another. Infection is usually transmitted by sexual contact when the moist, vulnerable mucous membrane tissues are in direct contact. However, one notable exception to this general rule is congenital syphilis–syphilis spread from the infected mother to her unborn child.

The Course of Untreated Syphilis

The sequelae of untreated syphilis are multiple and individually unpredictable. Infections may heal spontaneously or progress steadily to cause debilitation and death. Damage can include crippling, blindness, insanity, aortic insufficiency, visceral disorders, loss of nerve and muscle control, and the deterioration of bone and tissue. In addition, syphilis is often a secondary factor in the appearance of other infections and illnesses. Though there is a preponderance of reported complications within certain population groups, there is apparently no sex or ethnic group immune to the late sequelae of untreated syphilis. In the United States, the loss in manpower and the cost of institutional care of persons with syphilitic psychoses runs into millions of dollars annually. (If all syphilis infections were treated early, the occurrence of syphilitic psychoses would be prevented. Thus, this cost is in part an inverse measure of the efficiency of detection and treatment of syphilis in its early stages.) From observation, it is known that in certain individuals, untreated syphilis can result in serious disorders, but little information is available concerning the consequences of lack of therapy on a large number of infected persons in a homogeneous population. Probably the best statistical information available is based on two studies: the *Boeck-Bruusgaard* and the *Tuskegee.*

The Boeck-Bruusgaard Study

Between 1891 and 1910 Dr. Boeck, Professor of Dermatology and Venereology in the Oslo (Norway) Hospital, compiled medical records on the course of untreated syphilis in 1,978 persons admitted to his hospital with primary or secondary syphilis. He withheld treatment from them because of the inadequacy of available therapy; instead, they were hospitalized until symptoms disappeared. In 1929 Edvin Bruusgaard, his successor, compiled an analysis of the subsequent medical histories of 473 of these patients.[1] For years this study was one of the few available which provided information on the course of untreated syphilis, but, because of the small sample, its accuracy was questionable. A monumental restudy was conducted from 1948 to 1951 by Trygve Gjestland, who published his findings in a comprehensive monograph appearing in 1955.[2]

Of the 1,978 original patients, Gjestland studied 1,404, excluding only non-Norwegians and nonresidents of Oslo. Females outnumbered males approximately 2 to 1. The study group was comprised of persons living in the eastern section of the city, which at that time was the area of the underprivileged. Examination of the detailed clinical description of the symptoms of each person at the time of admission and during the course of stay at the hospital satisfied Gjestland that virtually all the diagnoses of syphilis were correct. Prior to conducting the study, he established several hypotheses to be tested and evaluated. Compilation of material was painstaking. Medical records were analyzed, living persons examined, and causes of deaths from death certificates tabulated. In a review by Clark and Danbolt, the following conclusions were drawn from Gjestland's monograph:

1. Although untreated syphilis was one of the causes of death in the sample, almost 90 percent of those in the sample died from other causes. The mortality rate from syphilis among males was twice that of females. Also, the nonfatal but debilitating effects of late complications (cardiovascular syphilis and neurosyphilis) affected males in

about the same ratio. Table 3.1 details causes of death among some of the original patients.

2. The mortality rate for all causes among untreated syphilitics in all age groups in the eastern zone was greater than that among nonsyphilitics from the same area. In addition, the mortality rates among all persons in the eastern zone were greater than those among residents of more prosperous areas of Oslo. These findings correspond with what demographers have long known to be true–that mortality rates among lower socioeconomic groups are higher than those among the better educated and more affluent segments of the population. However, Gjestland doubted that the higher death rates among syphilitics as compared to nonsyphilitics of the same peer group were attributable to syphilis. He postulated instead that within any group there were usually subgroups whose characteristics varied from those of the total sample.

3. Clinical secondary relapse is a common phenomenon in the prognosis of untreated syphilis. Observations were made on 1,035 patients admitted in a primary or secondary stage and known to have received no treatment. Of these, slightly less than 25 percent (244) relapsed to secondary symptoms within five years with most of the relapses occurring in the first year. Several of these people had multiple episodes of relapse. Lesions of the mouth, throat, and ano-genital region were involved in 85 percent of the cases.

Table 3.1   The Oslo study of untreated syphilis: primary causes of death by sex among 694 known dead

Primary causes of death	Males			Females		
	Number	Percent	Rank	Number	Percent	Rank
Tuberculosis	45	17.4	1	74	17.0	1
Syphilis	39	15.1	2	36	8.3	5
Cancer and other tumors	32	12.4	3	71	16.3	3
Diseases of circulatory system	28	10.8	4	72	16.6	2
Diseases of respiratory system	25	9.7	5	42	9.7	4
Sudden-unknown, unspecified	20	7.7	6	18	4.1	8
Diseases of urinary and genital tract	16	6.2	7	16	3.7	9
Diseases of nervous system and sense organs	14	5.4	8	34	7.8	6
Accidental deaths	11	4.2	9	9	2.1	10
Diseases of digestive system	7	2.7	10	24	5.5	7
All others	22	8.7		39	8.9	

Source: E. Gurney Clark and Niels Danbolt, "The Oslo Study of the Natural Course of Untreated Syphilis," The Medical Clinics of North America, 48, No. 3: 620 (May 1964).

4. "Spontaneous cure" is a term defying definition. Some authorities are very strict in interpreting the meaning of "cure"; others are more lenient. For a working definition, Gjestland suggests that a spontaneous cure can apply to anyone who, throughout life, experiences little or no inconvenience as a result of untreated syphilis. Using this criterion, he estimated that 60–70 out of every 100 untreated syphilitics cure spontaneously, a far higher percentage than is ordinarily suggested. However, the final outcome of syphilis in any individual cannot be predicted and can cause difficulties among 30–40 out of each 100 who remain untreated.[3]

Tuskegee Study

Further information on the course of untreated syphilis comes from the Tuskegee study of syphilitic Negro males in Macon County, Alabama.[4] This study, consisting of some 400 syphilitic patients and some 200 nonsyphilitic controls matched approximately by age, was begun in 1932 and is still under evaluation. Patients were selected for study on the basis of two reactive serologic tests for syphilis and the history of a primary lesion. Duration of infection varied from a few months to 72 years, with the majority having had their infections for more than 15 years. This group, then, includes only those who had survived their infections and had remained serologically reactive. Not fully known were the number of relapses, reinfections, and accidental treatments among the patients. But after taking into consideration these many factors, the following trends seem evident:

1. The expectation of life of individuals from ages 25 to 50 with syphilis was determined to be reduced by 17 percent.

2. General mortality rates for age-specific groups were higher among syphilitics than among the control group. After 20 years of follow-up, 40 percent of the syphilitics and 27 percent of the controls had died. After 30 years of follow-up, 59 percent of the syphilitics and 45 percent of the controls had died.

3. Most late sequelae involved the cardiovascular system, but neurosyphilis was not uncommon. Respiratory, genito-urinary, endocrine, and visceral complications among syphilitics were not significantly different from similar complications in the control group.

Both in this and in the Boeck study, mortality rates among syphilitics were higher than those of the general population. Neither study provides any definite explanation for this difference. Since today it is both undesirable and impossible to study the effects of untreated syphilis on a large and homogeneous population group, the Boeck-Bruusgaard and Tuskegee studies are possibly the best information on the long-term course of untreated syphilis we shall ever have.

Primary Syphilis

Primary syphilis is characterized by an initial lesion, called a chancre, which appears at the site of inoculation from ten to ninety days after exposure (average twenty-one days). The lesion is usually singular, and is most often found on the glans penis of the male and on the cervix of the female. After erosion, it presents a variety of forms, the most distinctive -- although not the most frequent -- being an indurated chancre. Such lesions are often undetected in the female because of their hidden location. Chancres are frequently accompanied by hard, nonfluctuant, painless, enlarged inguinal lymph nodes called satellite bubos. Primary lesions may also appear on the labia, scrotum, in the rectum or anus, in the mouth, or on the nipple. Chancres appear less frequently in these sites but often enough so that a complete and thorough physical examination should be made whenever syphilis is suspected.

The only absolute diagnosis for primary syphilis is a positive darkfield examination. A presumptive diagnosis can be based on a combination of the following factors -- exposure to an infected individual within three months, presence of indolent lesions, active or healing; a nonreactive spinal fluid; adenitis; and most important, a rapidly rising serologic titer. During the first week or more after the appearance of the lesion, the serologic tests for syphilis may remain negative. When a presumptive diagnosis is made, other venereal and nonvenereal genital infections should first be excluded. During the onset of primary stage symptoms, serologic tests are frequently nonreactive; because of this, a single, negative serologic test does not alone exclude infection. In all doubtful cases, at least two serologic tests for syphilis should be performed. Primary symptoms ordinarily disappear without treatment within three to five weeks. In untreated syphilis, the chancre frequently disappears spontaneously before the appearance of the secondary manifestations, but it may still be evident at the onset of the secondary stage.

Secondary Syphilis

Secondary symptoms generally appear six weeks to several months after infection and last anywhere from a few days to a year before disappearing. These symptoms usually appear as involution of the primary chancre occurs, but there may be an indeterminate asymptomatic period between the two stages. Manifestations include a local or generalized cutaneous rash, condylomata lata of the ano-genital region, malaise, fever, alopecia, mucous patches of the mouth, and a reactive serologic test. Spinal fluid examinations are positive in about 25 percent of secondary cases.[5] Skin lesions may be macular, papular, papulosquamous, or pustular, but never vesicular or bulbous in adults as they sometimes are in early congenital syphilis in infants. The lesions are seldom pruritic; they are bilateral and symmetrical. As a rule, *T. pallidum* may be demonstrated from any mucous or cutaneous secondary lesion, but most easily from a moist one. However, failure to demonstrate the spirochete in suspect lesions does not rule out a diagnosis of secondary syphilis. Alopecia and condylomata lata are less common than cutaneous lesions. Malaise and fever are more likely to develop when systemic reactions to infection are pronounced.

Relapse and Reinfection

Infectious syphilis includes the primary, secondary, and early latent stages. During the stage of early latency, the untreated and, perhaps, the inadequately treated patient will have periodic relapses to the secondary types of lesions followed by spontaneous healing. This relapsing tendency occurs for the most part during the first two years of infection. Often immunologic changes occur which prevent the appearance of infectious skin lesions but not the progression of the organism in other body tissues. Thus, while the stages of primary and secondary syphilis may be regarded as continuously infectious, early latent syphilis is intermittently so, depending upon relapse.

For years many authorities have believed there is no natural or induced immunity to syphilis. This has not yet been disproven, but considerable evidence exists that suggests resistance to infection in some individuals. Clinic records throughout the United States contain case histories of many contacts who have been repeatedly exposed to lesion syphilis but who never develop any clinical or serological signs of infection. Other information has been compiled indicating that one infection, whether treated or untreated, may produce strong resistance to subsequent infection in some individuals.

However, following cure of early syphilis, reinfection does frequently occur. Apparently because of physiologic changes resulting from the original infection, many reinfections are asymptomatic and are characterized only by changes in serologic reactivity. The difficulty of detecting reinfections and distinguishing them from relapses or treatment failures may explain why few are diagnosed as such.

Shortly after penicillin was introduced to syphilis therapy, several studies were conducted in an attempt to determine accurate criteria for distinguishing between relapses and reinfections. These studies were initiated after numerous reports of what at first appeared to be treatment failures among patients treated with penicillin. Reinfection had long been believed to be a relatively rare phenomenon, even though no reliable methods existed for distinguishing between initial infections, relapses, and reinfection. After reviewing the literature, Beerman concluded that reinfection was possibly more common than previously suspected, but that there was no accurate method of diagnosis.[6] In 1948 Schamberg and Steiger found that many apparent treatment failures were in actuality due to "ping-pong" infections, i.e., reinfections from an untreated steady sex partner such as a wife or girl friend.[7] However, they too were unable to develop an infallible method for distinguishing relapses from reinfections. The problem remains unsolved to the present day. The principal significance of such a decision lies in the fact that a reinfection is treated exactly as a new case, whereas a relapse may require increased antibiotic therapy on retreatment if a low dosage schedule was used initially.

One of the most carefully controlled investigations into syphilis immunity and inoculation was undertaken in a special study of a prison population. In 1952 the Public Health Service, in cooperation with the New York State Department of Health and the Department of Correction, conducted a syphilis inoculation study among sixty-two male volunteers confined in Sing-Sing Prison.[8] Clinical, laboratory, and anamnestic data were compiled on each of the patients before attempts at inoculation began. Fifty-four of the sixty-two volunteers had verified histories of previously treated syphilis; the eight prisoners who served as control patients had no history or evidence of infection. As the study progressed, clinical observations and notes were made, color photographs of lesions and suspicious dermatological conditions were taken, and blood specimens were drawn periodically to be evaluated with the New York State Complement Fixation Test and the *Treponema Pallidum* Immobilization Test. Experiments were conducted with both heat-killed and virulent strains of *T. pallidum*. At the end of four months, all the patients received six million units of penicillin (PAM) in five equal doses as curative treatment. The careful planning, close observation, and control of this study made its findings as conclusive as any in the area of syphilis inoculation. No attempt will be made to summarize the procedures involved in the experiment, but a few of the tentative conclusions are worth presenting. Because of the small sample of patients, however, some of the findings are not necessarily conclusive.

1. Nichol's strain of *T. pallidum*, taken from rabbits in which it had been maintained since 1912, retained its virulence for man.

2. Using the Nichol's strain of *T. pallidum*, infection through inoculation in the human host is definitely possible. The greater the concentration of treponemes in the inoculum, the greater is the chance of infection and the more likely the rapid appearance of symptoms.

3. Not all patients who were inoculated produced lesions. Of those with lesions, not all were typical, nor were all darkfield positive.

4. Although injections of heat-killed treponemes induced varying serologic responses among previously infected prisoners, no changes in circulating antibodies were demonstrated in nonsyphilitic control patients given the same antigen. These findings appear to decrease the possibility of an immunizing vaccine using heat-killed *T. pallidum*.

5. Persons diagnosed with syphilis in late latent, neurological, and congenital stages before inoculation was attempted were those most resistant to infection. In a general way, this reaction was influenced by the duration of their original infection prior to treatment. However, the phenomenon of immunity was not proven.

The studies and investigations previously outlined support the following general conclusions:

1. Although its frequency is unknown, reinfection occurs.

2. Resistance to reinfection may develop in some individuals. Immunity to reinfection is not established.

3. Infection by inoculation of human beings with virulent *T. pallidum* is possible, both in nonsyphilitic persons and in those previously treated for syphilis.

4. Initial infections, reinfections, and relapses may vary in clinical appearance and in the serologic response induced, but not consistently or predictably. Without other information the actual category of infection cannot be conclusively diagnosed.

For control purposes it makes little difference whether a lesion case represents a relapse, a reinfection, or an initial infection. All are accompanied by lesions and must be treated to prevent transmission to other persons. Immunity is still a matter of concern in syphilis control and is presently being studied, but no method of artificially producing immunity to infection has yet been developed.

Diagnosis of Latent Syphilis Both Early and Late

Latent syphilis, by definition, is hidden syphilis. There are no clinical manifestations of the disease. A diagnosis usually is established on the basis of reactive serologic tests after the possibilities of other stages of syphilis have been ruled out by physical and spinal fluid examination.

A history of exposure, genital lesions, or cutaneous eruptions may be used to establish a diagnosis. In the absence of other signs and symptoms, a reactive serologic test must be considered diagnostic of latent syphilis until the reaction is proved to be caused by something else. The spinal fluid examination in latent syphilis must be nonreactive.

Latency is arbitrarily divided into two stages, early latent and late latent. No true line may be drawn between the two stages, because the disease is a continuum, and its progress depends very largely on the physiology of the infected individual. The *International Lists of Diseases and Causes of Death* defines early latent syphilis as asymptomatic syphilis of less than four years' duration. In the past few years, there has been a trend in the United States to define early latency as syphilis of less than one year's duration, for it is during this time that infection is of greatest epidemiological and medical significance. The early latent period, then, begins when secondary symptoms disappear and ends one to four years after the infection was contracted, depending upon the definition used. (A brief period of latency may also occur during an indeterminate asymptomatic period between primary and secondary stages. How frequently this occurs is unknown.)

When the early latent period ends, the late latent period begins and continues throughout life, except in those individuals who progress to late symptomatic stages.

Late Syphilis

Late syphilis is a general term, including asymptomatic and symptomatic neurosyphilis, cardiovascular syphilis, and late benign (visceral gumma, osseous, and cutaneous) syphilis. The enumerated categories of late syphilis are not infectious, except to the fetus. Serologic tests and spinal fluid examinations are usually reactive.

Late syphilis lesions are chronic and destructive. Late manifestations include crippling, blindness, insanity (paresis), aortic insufficiency, and death.

Congenital Syphilis

Congenital syphilis is acquired *in utero* by the developing fetus and is active at birth. If lesions are present, congenital syphilis may be diagnosed by darkfield examination; serologic tests are reactive in all cases. Most of the serious damage from untreated congenital syphilis becomes evident in later years. In past years eye damage eventually occurred in about 80 percent of all untreated cases.[9] Imperfect development and uneven spacing of teeth, poor bone structure, hydrarthrosis of joints, facial scars, and deafness are less common but still are significant sequelae. About two-thirds of all living children born to diseased mothers will be infected with congenital syphilis. The untreated congenital syphilitic has a higher mortality rate than the general population and is likely to suffer impairment from his infection at some time during his life.

Congenital syphilis results only from acquired, untreated infection in the mother. Untreated maternal syphilis produces not only living syphilitic offspring but a high proportion of abortions and stillbirths as well. Figures compiled before World War II indicate that stillbirths are eight times more frequent in infected mothers than in the population at large.[10] Estimates of the percentage of pregnancies terminated by abortions and/or stillbirths run from about 24 percent (Kampmeier) to 46 percent (McKelvey and Turner, cited by Stokes).

These figures were compiled in the days before penicillin therapy, generally on small samples of clinic patients among whom health standards were low and morbidity indices for all diseases high.

Today congenital syphilis is a medical rarity. Better health and nutrition through prenatal care and effective treatment when infection does occur have combined to eradicate almost all congenital syphilis infections. In recent years they have comprised less than 0.00008 percent of all live births. Still, if a mother is infected and remains untreated, the probability of producing a healthy, uninfected child is slight.

Laboratory Procedures in Syphilis Diagnosis

Darkfield examinations

The only absolute diagnosis of syphilis is a positive darkfield examination. This procedure is a microscopic examination of exudate from a lesion or rash suspected of being syphilitic. A compound microscope with a darkfield condenser is used for the performance of this test. The result is such that objects are illuminated by reflected light against a dark background or field. A positive diagnosis can be made by a trained physician on the basis of characteristic morphology and motility. Conventional brightfield techniques cannot be used because the staining and fixing procedures involved would kill the spirochete, precluding the motility which is essential for accurate diagnosis. Since darkfield examinations must be made from suspicious lesions or rashes, they can only be performed during the following stages of infection: primary, secondary, early congenital, and infectious relapse. Positive findings are diagnostic. Failure to demonstrate the organisms from the suspected lesion after repeated examinations may mean that (1) the lesion is not syphilitic, (2) the patient has received systemic or local treatment, (3) too much time has elapsed since the appearance of the lesion, or (4) the lesion may be of late syphilis.

If findings remain negative, the patient should be asked to return the next day for further examination. Only after extensive study has failed to reveal any *T. pallida* should a negative report be issued. The general practice is to have a darkfield performed daily for three consecutive days, and if the darkfield is still negative on the third day, the patient is followed serologically. In situations where it is not feasible to ask the patient to return, prophylactic treatment may be advisable on the basis of clinical judgment of the appearance of the lesion, history, and epidemiologic data. When all examinations over a period of time are negative, the decision to treat or not to treat must be made by the individual physician after consideration of all other available evidence.

Serologic testing

Unlike the darkfield examination, a positive serologic test is presumptive evidence of syphilis, but, like the darkfield, a negative test does not exclude the possibility of infection. Despite these limitations, both positive and negative results still have significance and are among the most important considerations in the differential diagnosis of syphilis. So valuable are the results from standard serologic tests performed by trained personnel that public health laws in many states require the performance of at least one test before a diagnosis of syphilis is made. A repeated positive blood test makes the diagnosis probable, and if the history and physical and epidemiologic data are added, the diagnosis of syphilis can be confirmed by a positive laboratory test. Tests can be performed on specimens of spinal fluid or tissue exudate; these results can be very important, though not always essential, to accurate diagnosis.

Serologic tests vary according to stage. In primary syphilis, blood tests may be reactive; however, they can be negative at the time of treatment and reactive shortly thereafter. This is a result of the length of time necessary for body defenses to produce a detectable amount of antibody to infection. In primary syphilis, the blood titer will almost always descend to a nonreactive level within six months after treatment. In secondary syphilis, blood titers are generally quite high and may remain so for several months after treatment. In most cases the serologic titer will become non-reactive within two years. In a few situations an individual may retain seropositivity for several years or even for life. In early latent, late latent, and late congenital syphilis, blood titers are generally low before treatment and may change little afterward. It is not unusual for individuals treated in any of these stages to remain seropositive for life. The longer the duration of infection, the greater the probability of life-long serologic reactivity.

In the sixty years which have elapsed since serologic examinations were first introduced to syphilis management, a number of tests have been developed. Several studies have been conducted on the reliability of these tests, and while some variation among them exists, those in use today are generally sensitive to and specific for syphilis. There are two general types of serologic tests: Nontreponemal (those employing lipid or cardiolipin antigens) and treponemal (those using either *T. pallidum* or the nonvirulent Reiter treponeme as antigen). Nontreponemal tests are fast, inexpensive, and widely used; treponemal tests are often avoided by laboratories because of the time and expense involved.

Nontreponemal (Reagin) Tests. Nontreponemal tests are designed for the detection of an antibody-like substance called reagin found in the serum of an infected patient and thought to be caused by the interaction of *T. pallidum* with body tissue. There are several nontreponemal tests in use today, which are basically of two types: (1) flocculation tests and (2) complement fixation tests. Flocculation tests include VDRL (Venereal Disease Research Laboratory), Kline, Kahn, Hinton, and Mazzini; complement fixation tests are fewer, with only the Kolmer commonly employed today. The Wassermann test, the original serologic test for syphilis, was a complement fixation test but is no longer in use.

1. Flocculation Tests (qualitative and quantitative): Flocculation is a reaction in which a suspension of antigen particles, when added to serum, plasma, or spinal fluid specimens containing antibody, will form discrete, usually visible clumps or floccules. Serologically, this type of test can be performed either microscopically or macroscopically and is reported as reactive, weakly reactive, or nonreactive. When any degree of reactivity is obtained in the screening (qualitative) test, a quantitative test should be performed. Quantitative evaluation of specimens is helpful because a base line of reactivity is established from which changes can be measured. Such a test is conducted by diluting the serum, usually in a geometric progression, until an end point of reactivity is reached.

EXAMPLE:

Serum dilution	1:1	1:2	1:4	1:8	1:16	1:32	1:64	1:128
Test reading	R	R	R	R	R	R	WR	NR

This result would be reported as reactive 1:32 or 32 dils because 32 is the end point of reactivity (64 is the point of weak reactivity and at 128 there is no reactivity). In general, titers are higher in secondary syphilis and late symptomatic syphilis than in other stages. With latent syphilis, titers may be high but are usually low or moderate. For public health purposes titers of 1:8 or above are significant because they most often accompany an infectious stage.

Once a specimen has demonstrated any degree of reactivity, subsequent specimens should be evaluated using the same test as the original. A battery of tests is no longer recommended and is of little value since results from one test cannot be accurately correlated with results from another. Using a single test, a falling, rising, or stable titer can provide some help to a physician in determining the significance of an infection. If results are inconclusive and diagnosis remains a problem, use of another test is acceptable.

2. Complement Fixation Tests: Complement fixation takes place when an active complement (a lytic substance in normal serum), an antigen, and its antibody are brought together under the proper temperature and time conditions. The addition of an indicator system permits the results to be read macroscopically. Like flocculation tests, complement fixation tests may be performed either qualitatively or quantitatively. With the exception of the New York State Complement Fixation test, quantitative findings are reported in terms of the highest dilution giving a reactive result (see previous example). Complement fixation tests require more exacting techniques, more time, and elaborate laboratory equipment without offering the advantage of greater specificity. For this reason many laboratories have discontinued the use of these tests, and as faster, cheaper, and more reliable techniques are developed, they will probably continue to diminish in popularity.

3. Rapid Reagin Tests: Rapid Reagin Tests are special purpose tests using flocculation procedures on plasma or unheated serum. They are used as rough screening procedures in situations where large numbers of specimens are tested and speed is essential. Specimens reacting to these tests should be further evaluated with other more specific tests. Examples are the RPR (Rapid Plasma Reagin) test, which has been used in screening programs on the Mexican border; the RPR Teardrop Card test, a procedure designed for field use in jail testing and migrant farm labor screening programs, but which is now more widely used in clinics for immediate results; and the RPR Circle Card test, a method used primarily in laboratories. The USR (Unheated Serum Reagin) and PCT (Plasmacrit) tests are two rapid reagin tests which are widely used in hospital, laboratory, and blood bank screening procedures.

Treponemal Tests. Treponemal tests are tests for the detection of treponemal antibody produced in response to syphilitic infection. Though not 100 percent sensitive in detecting old infections, treponemal tests are more specific than nontreponemal tests and are used primarily in resolving diagnostic problem cases. When diagnosis must be made solely through the use of a serologic test, a treponemal test is the type which should be used.

1. *Treponema Pallidum* Immobilization Test: The TPI test employs the causative agent of syphilis as the antigen. When serum containing antibody to *T. pallidum* combines with antigen and active complement, *T. pallidum* is immobilized. Tests are read microscopically and are reported as reactive, weakly reactive, and nonreactive.

2. FTA (Fluorescent Treponemal Antibody) Tests: The FTA tests employ virulent Nichol's strain of *T. pallidum* as the antigen. The FTA-200 is the most common modification in use. A complicated series of procedures allows the technician to determine the fluorescence or nonfluorescence of *T. pallidum* under a U-V microscope. Results of FTA tests are reported as either reactive or nonreactive.

3. Newly developed and currently under evaluation is the FTA-ABS (absorption) test. The same principles are involved as in the FTA tests except that antigens common for other treponemes (such as *T. microdentia* and *Borrelia refringens*) are absorbed from the specimen, leaving only the specific *T. pallidum* antigen if it is present. This test shows promise because it is as highly specific as the TPI test and more sensitive than the FTA-200.

4. Kolmer Test with the Reiter Protein Antigen (KRP Test): The KRP is another of the treponemal tests, but one which uses the nonvirulent Reiter-Treponeme cultivated *in vitro*. The KRP is sometimes referred to as the RPCF (Reiter Protein Complement Fixation) test and is alone among tests which can be performed by either treponemal or nontreponemal techniques. The techniques for the KRP are the same as those for the nontreponemal Kolmer test except for the antigen. The KRP is fairly specific but lacks sensitivity.

Some of the tests used for serologic testing can also be adapted to spinal fluid examinations. These can be performed with nontreponemal antigen tests such as the VDRL and Kolmer. Results are reported numerically when a quantitative test is conducted. A spinal fluid examination is a valuable adjunct in the diagnosis of syphilis infection; false positive reactions are rare, and a reactive result is virtually diagnostic of past or present central nervous system syphilis. Spinal fluid examinations also include a cell count and a total protein determination. An increased cell count, increased total protein, and reactive spinal fluid examination are highly indicative of active neurosyphilis.

The Biologic False Positive (BFP) Reactions. Positive results from serologic tests would be 100 percent diagnostic of syphilis infection but for one infrequent, but important, phenomenon: the biologic false positive reaction. A biologic false positive reaction is defined as a reactive (or positive) serologic test for syphilis which in actuality is not caused by syphilis. These reactions are due to the inherent nature of serologic tests, for they detect not *T. pallidum* but reagin, an antibody-like substance in normal serum thought to be produced in response to infection. Most reagin responses are caused by syphilis, but some result from other infections such as lupus erythematosus, infectious mononucleosis, hepatitis, malaria, and rheumatic fever. Cancer, narcotics addiction, pregnancy, and even smallpox vaccination are thought to sometimes account for reactive blood tests.

The probability of false positive reactions in random samples of sera from presumably nonsyphilitic individuals has been estimated in several studies. Moore suggested that one in every three to five thousand healthy, normal individuals presumably free from syphilis and other diseases known to cause biologic false positive reactions may have a reactive serologic test for syphilis.[11]

Eagle, after testing sera from 40,000 white college students, postulated that in healthy persons apparently free from syphilis, about one in 4,000 (.025 percent) will have a false positive reaction.[12] Kolmer and Lynch compiled figures for false positive reactions with tests employing eight different cardiolipin antigens. Such reactions occurred in 4 of 2,523 specimens (.16 percent).[13] Since the positive results in this study were not verified by the TPI, about half of them could be considered syphilitic in origin, reducing the true number of false reactions to about .08 percent. This compares favorably with the .025 percent observed in Eagle's study.

These studies are not conclusive, but they do indicate that the BFP is quite uncommon and certainly more the exception than the rule. A positive serologic test is most often indicative of past or present syphilitic infection and should be so considered until proven otherwise.

Nontreponemal antigen tests may be supplemented by treponemal immobilization, agglutination, or fluorescent antibody tests to aid in the diagnosis of biologic false positive reactions. These supplemental tests along with a complete history, physical examination, dates and results of past and present serologic tests, and any indicated spinal fluid results should lead to the proper diagnosis and management of the overwhelming majority of patients.

Treatment

Penicillin is the drug of choice for the treatment of all stages of syphilis. It is usually administered by intramuscular injection, with half of the total dosage administered in any one session being given in each buttock. The Public Health Service recommends the following treatment schedules by stage of syphilis:

Primary or Secondary. (a) 2.4 million units of benzathine penicillin G in one session; *or*

(b) 4.8 million units of procaine penicillin G with 2 percent aluminum monostearate (PAM): 2.4 million units at the first session and 1.2 million units at each of two subsequent sessions, three days apart; *or*

(c) 4.8 million units of aqueous procaine penicillin G with 600,000 units given daily for eight days; *or*

(d) alternate antibiotics.

Treat according to stage. No additional medicine is necessary.

Latent (both Early and Late). (a) With a nonreactive spinal fluid, 2.4 million units of benzathine penicillin G in one session; without a spinal fluid examination, treatment must encompass the possibility of asymptomatic neurosyphilis: 3.0 million units of benzathine penicillin G in each of two sessions, seven days apart, for a total of 6.0 million units is adequate; *or*

(b) 4.8 million units of PAM: 2.4 million units in one session and 1.2 million units in each of two subsequent sessions, seven days apart; *or*

(c) 4.8 million units of aqueous procaine penicillin G: 600,000 units daily for eight days; *or*

(d) alternate antibiotics. When patient sensitivity to penicillin precludes the use of this drug, then erythromycin, tetracycline, chlortetracycline, oxytetracycline, and demethylchlortetracycline are the best alternate choices.

Late Syphilis (includes neurosyphilis, cardiovascular syphilis, and late benign syphilis). (a) 6.0 to 9.0 million units of benzathine penicillin G given 3.0 million units at sessions seven days apart; *or*

(b) 6.0 to 9.0 million units of PAM given 1.2 million units per session at three-day intervals; *or*

(c) 6.0 to 9.0 million units of aqueous procaine penicillin G, 600,000 units daily. Any benefit from more than 10 million units has not been demonstrated.

Syphilis in Pregnancy. Treat according to stage. No additional medication is necessary. Retreatment is indicated if there is any doubt concerning adequacy of previous treatment.

Early Congenital (under two years of age). (a) 50,000 units of benzathine penicillin G per kilogram of body weight in a single injection; *or*

(b) 100,000 units of aqueous procaine penicillin G per kilogram (or 50,000 per lb.) of body weight divided into daily dosages over a ten-day period.

Late Congenital (over two years of age). In treating children under twelve years of age, treatment dosages should be adjusted for weight as in early congenital syphilis. In treating persons twelve years of age or older but weighing more than 70 pounds: (a) if spinal fluid is reactive, treat as neurosyphilis; *or*

(b) if spinal fluid is nonreactive, treat as late latent syphilis.

All patients should be carefully examined, followed, and treated on an individual basis.

In cases of penicillin sensitivity, broad spectrum antibiotics may be used. Erythromycin is the most effective of these, and tetracycline has produced good results in some cases. Neither is fully evaluated, but apparently they are more effective than any other alternate antibiotic.

Oral antibiotics should be avoided whenever possible. They are not as effective as intramuscular shots and by nature are fraught with built-in nonmedical problems. Patients often forget to take tablets or decide not to take them. In several known case histories, patients have sold their medicine to finance alcohol or narcotics. Oral preparations are acceptable if they are administered on the spot with adequate supervision to insure ingestion. Otherwise, they should be avoided.

Anaphylactic reactions and deaths have occurred following the use of penicillin. Anaphylactic reactions may be anticipated by observing symptoms such as vertigo, nausea, flushing, itching, or even abdominal pain. Such reactions are extremely rare but emergency measures should be immediately available whenever penicillin is administered. When there is a history of any serious allergy, penicillin should be administered only with the greatest caution. A previous reaction to penicillin should preclude its use.

The Jarisch-Herxheimer reaction is presumably caused by the rapid killing of many treponemes. It consists of a transient fever that may or may not be associated with a temporary exacerbation of syphilitic lesions. The reaction, as a rule, occurs within twelve hours following the first dose of a potent treponemicidal agent. The reaction is common following the onset of treatment of early syphilis, but it is frequently unnoticed by the patient. Following treatment of late syphilis, Herxheimer reactions are rarely noted except in general paresis, but this is not cause for stopping treatment.

Prognosis after penicillin therapy is excellent except in those cases of long duration where substantial damage has already taken place. After treatment no further deterioration due to active disease will occur, and if the initial recommended dosage is used, few cases will require retreatment. Penicillin is the most efficacious treatment available today. Mercury, arsenic, and bismuth are obsolete and have no place in modern syphilis management.

4 / Venereal Disease Casefinding and Control Measures in the Twentieth Century

The history of venereal disease control prior to the twentieth century is a history of continual improvisation, quackery, and failure. Before arsenicals were discovered, effective treatment for syphilis was simply not available, and the various techniques and agents employed as therapy served at best to reduce symptoms. Epidemiologic control through the use of quarantines was often attempted. While sound in theory, the procedure was in most cases ineffective, for little short of solitary confinement can effectively isolate an infected person from other individuals. But with the advent of arsenicals in 1910, the quest for an effective treatment for syphilis, sought in vain for four centuries, finally reached its objective.

Despite the availability of therapy, control efforts at first elicited little sympathy or public support. Syphilis was so taboo that there was resistance to recognizing the problem officially. Indication of the atmosphere is revealed in a 1908 memorandum from the Treasury Department in response to a request made by the Public Health Service to publish a pamphlet on venereal disease: "The matter contained in this bulletin is not in keeping with the dignity of the fiscal department of government."

The toleration of the status quo expressed in this memorandum did not long endure after the results of serologic testing and physical examination of enlistees during World War I became known. These results indicated that about 5.6 percent of all persons examined had evidence of some type of venereal infection.[1] Until this time, no national measures had been taken to deal with the problem. However, it was now apparent that venereal disease constituted a health problem of major proportions, and Congress took action.

The Chamberlain-Kahn Act of 1918 was significant in that it set a precedent for dealing with venereal disease in a coordinated manner on a national level. The bill created the Division of Venereal Disease within the Public Health Service to provide consultation and information about the establishment and operation of programs in each state. Cash grants-in-aid for program operation were also provided. With the passage of this bill, assistance from a national agency became available on request to state and local health departments choosing to combat venereal disease problems in their jurisdiction. Most state control programs placed emphasis on the medical treatment of existing infections, on the principle that by rendering cases noninfectious, spread of disease would diminish and the overall syphilis reservoir could be reduced. It was hoped that eventually control would be achieved.

Unfortunately, interest in venereal disease control waned after World War I, and though the bill remained in effect, there was little effort to promote venereal disease control and eradication as a public health responsibility. In 1936 Thomas Parran, former Chief of the Venereal Disease Division, became Surgeon General of the Public Health Service, and in this position he was instrumental in generating renewed interest in syphilis control. Newspapers carried numerous articles concerning syphilis; lectures by health authorities were given; Parran himself discussed the problem on the radio. His book *Shadow on the Land* dramatized the danger and cost of untreated syphilis.[2]

Attitudes gradually changed, and in 1938 Congress passed the La Follette-Bulwinkle Bill, the act which is the basis of the present national control program. Like its predecessor twenty years earlier, this bill provided funds for the operation of local programs, but it allowed for the expansion of the Venereal Disease Division in order to improve research, treatment schedules, patient follow-up, record keeping, and program analysis. The introduction of sulfonamides to gonorrhea therapy in 1937 enabled the program to provide assistance to the many communities where gonorrhea was a problem. However, the major emphasis remained on syphilis.

In the years prior to and during World War II, many of the public health laws which are today an integral part of venereal disease control were enacted and put into effect. In 1935 Connecticut became the first state to require premarital blood tests for both males and females; in 1938 Rhode Island passed the first state law requiring prenatal blood tests in pregnant women. Laboratory reactor reporting laws were passed in some states; in others, laws requiring the reporting of syphilis and/or gonorrhea were also passed. In addition to these laws voluntary screening and control measures were taken in the form of pre-employment examinations, blood donor screening, and routine serologic testing on hospital admission. These measures helped bring to treatment thousands of cases which might otherwise have remained undetected, and treatment on a large scale was carried on throughout the country.

At the start of World War II the demands of rapid mobilization led directly to a number of new and more effective processes for venereal disease control. Some of these processes are the conceptual bases for present-day operations.

Prior to this mass induction process, public health officials had recognized that rapid mass movement could spread venereal disease throughout the world. As a result, some 15 million men entering the Armed Services either as volunteers or through the Selective Service System were carefully examined. Three-quarters of a million had positive serologic tests for syphilis and/or clinical signs or symptoms. Over 300,000 of the infected men were treated rapidly by civilian health departments, rendered noninfectious, and inducted into the Armed Services.

During World War II, venereal disease rates among the military continued to cause major problems in reduced efficiency and lost time. An immediate need for better control and faster treatment was apparent. The Eight Point Agreement, a control plan whereby the military services and civilian agencies worked in close cooperation with the Public Health Service in the follow-up of contacts to infectious syphilis and the suppression of prostitution and vice, was implemented.

Prostitutes and other contacts to military personnel were treated as inpatients in newly organized Rapid Treatment Centers on new, shorter treatment schedules ranging from one day to several weeks. These schedules were also employed on members of the military. While far from perfect, they were a considerable improvement over the old 18-month schedules and partially resolved the difficult task of rapidly treating large numbers of individuals whose immediate services were vital. Nevertheless, venereal disease remained a major military health problem.

The centuries-old quest for effective, rapid treatment for syphilis ended in 1943 when Dr. John Mahoney demonstrated the efficacy of penicillin as syphilis therapy. A year later he and his associates developed a suitable schedule for the treatment of gonorrhea. Until the end of the war, difficulties in the production and refinement of penicillin limited its use primarily to the military, but within the military services, venereal infections ceased to be significant health problems. Although the acquisition of disease continued at a high level, lost time and debility from infections were drastically reduced.

Syphilis control in the civilian population became a practical reality with the development of effective penicillin therapy immediately after World War II. Up until 1947 emphasis had been placed upon control laws, development of treatment, establishment of clinics and treatment centers, and provision of grants to operate these facilities. Because of the inadequacy of therapy and the large number of persons undergoing long-term arsenical treatment, syphilis control of necessity was based on caseholding rather than casefinding. After the war ended, penicillin became widely available for civilian use, eliminating the caseholding problem and making feasible control programs designed to detect the thousands of unknown and untreated infections comprising the syphilis reservoir.

Mass testing of virtually total populations became the casefinding method of choice. During the ten-year period following World War II, state and local health departments throughout the United States diagnosed and treated over two and one-quarter million persons with syphilis. In addition, a substantial number of persons previously treated were re-treated with penicillin during these surveys.

The decreasing yields from a cost effectiveness standpoint and the development of alternative casefinding techniques brought an end to mass blood testing activity. As mass testing was eliminated, selective testing of suspected high incidence subgroups of the population was initiated. Blood testing of these groups, predetermined primarily by epidemiologic investigation, replaced mass testing. Although employed only on a limited basis today, selective testing is still productive in testing agricultural migrant labor and inmates of jails or penal institutions. Thus, the very success of selective testing contributed to its limited use. The low yields, generally less than one percent brought to treatment in recent years, has resulted in the use of other more productive casefinding methods centering around the diagnosed infectious case.

By the mid-1950's reported cases of syphilis had declined so sharply that this disease was considered another conquered health problem. As a result, federal funds to states were decreased, clinics were practically eliminated, and epidemiologic follow-up was all but abandoned. New preparations of penicillin made it possible to treat syphilis rapidly and effectively on an outpatient basis. Because syphilis appeared to be nearly eliminated, many felt that syphilis control programs were no longer necessary, and attention was focused on a gonorrhea control program.

Prior to 1952, gonorrhea control consisted largely of the diagnosis and treatment of the infected individual. In 1952 the Public Health Service, with the cooperation of state and large city health departments, launched the first major attempt to control gonorrhea. The program was called "Speed-Zone Epidemiology."

Mahoney and his associates had demonstrated that the incubation period of experimentally acquired gonorrhea in males ranged up to 31 days, but that 85 percent of the infections produced clinical symptoms within 6 days.[3] The productive targets for epidemiologic investigation appeared to be sex contacts of male gonococcal urethritis patients exposed within the period beginning 6 days prior to the onset of clinical symptoms and ending at the time of volunteering at the clinic. Penicillin in aluminum monostearate appeared to protect the patient from reinfection for a minimal period of 72 hours. Because reinfection from the same source is frequent, rapid investigation of contacts must be completed within the penicillin protection period of 72 hours in order to minimize reinfection. Speed-zone epidemiology projects operated in 19 cities from 1952 to 1958. In most cities the ultimate objective of a significant reduction in male volunteers was not accomplished. However, the intermediate objective of examination and treatment of a significant number of female contacts was accomplished. In 1963 Thayer and Moore indicated that treatment failures in females ranged from 20-40 percent of those females treated in a cooperative clinical study, suggesting that this factor appeared to be the reason for no significant reduction in male gonorrhea cases.[4]

The apparent victory over syphilis was also brief. From 1958 to 1965 there was a continuing rise in reported early infectious syphilis case rates to over three times the 1957 level. In 1966 the number of such cases decreased slightly. The slight increases noted in 1958 and 1959 were at first believed to have little significance, but the additional increase noted in 1960 indicated that a resurgence in infectious syphilis had occurred.

The increase in reported cases of primary and secondary syphilis was related to the epidemiologic investigation of individual cases of infectious syphilis and the follow-up of reactive serologic tests reported by public and private laboratories. These two methods are the principal ways in which all new cases are brought to treatment by health departments today.

FOLLOW-UP OF SEROLOGIC TESTS

Of the 22,473 primary and secondary syphilis cases reported in fiscal year 1966, 29 percent were brought to treatment as a result of the rapid follow-up of persons with a reactive serologic test for syphilis.

Although these persons had clinical evidence of early syphilis, their reactive serologies were discovered through several areas of routine testing—such as premarital, prenatal, and pre-employment—and not because they sought medical attention on their own. Since their signs and symptoms did not alert them sufficiently to seek diagnosis, rapid follow-up of reactors was essential in bringing these persons to treatment. This situation was also demonstrated in nationwide studies in 1948 and 1963 in which 55 to 78 percent of persons brought to treatment through the follow-up of reactive serologies admitted that they had recognized signs or symptoms but did not seek medical attention.[5, 6]

Although many states employed the follow-up of reactive serologic tests as a means of surveillance in the early years of the program, not until mid-1962 was a national, relatively uniform follow-up program instituted by the Public Health Service. Reactor programs are a surveillance detection measure necessitated primarily by the failure of hospitals and private physicians to report all cases of syphilis and by the failure of a significant number of individuals to seek treatment during symptomatic stages.

Reactor follow-up serves as a morbidity reporting device for primary, secondary, and early latent cases upon which epidemiological activity can be initiated. By means of epidemiologic investigation of infectious syphilis cases resulting from reactor follow-up, health departments are in a position to prevent the further spread of infection.

In the United States there are approximately 9,200 public and private laboratories performing 38,000,000 serologic examinations annually, of which 1,149,000 are estimated to be reactive. Current program data show that approximately 709,000 or 62 percent of these reactors are reported. In 31 states and the District of Columbia, laws or health department regulations require that laboratories performing serologic tests report reactive results. In states without such laws, some laboratories report reactors voluntarily. The Public Health Service strongly recommends that notification of positive tests be required in all states. In recent years several states have passed such laws, and analysis of results indicates that reporting of reactive serologies by private laboratories increased 15 to 20 percent and by public laboratories as much as 7 percent.

However, in states both with and without reactor notification laws, the number of reactors reported does not, as previously mentioned, represent the total reactor population. Some laboratories may choose to ignore regulations, or physicians may send specimens to private laboratories in states without reporting laws. When this occurs, it is difficult to determine the total number of reactors. An estimated 440,000 reactors remain unreported annually, and the enactment of notification laws or regulations in those states where they are not in effect would tend to increase the overall effectiveness of the control program.

In the face of a rising reported incidence of syphilis in the United States since 1957, the Public Health Service recommends the continuance of routine serologic testing programs. However, for any serologic testing activity to be effective in casefinding in the United States, it is essential that the notification of reactive serologic tests to appropriate health authorities be required by law in all states. Only then can routine serologic testing serve as both a surveillance and a casefinding tool

Routine Serologic Testing Programs and Examinations

Premarital Examinations

A review of marriage laws in the United States indicates that five states have no legal requirement concerning syphilis premarital examinations.[7] The other forty-five states require that marriage applicants have blood tests and physical examinations for syphilis.

Thousands of cases of syphilis have been detected as a result of premarital blood testing since the testing program began in the late 1930's. Since World War II the reduction of the syphilis reservoir has reduced the yield from premarital tests, but they remain a valuable surveillance measure for detecting sporadic cases.

Specific figures for syphilis cases brought to treatment as a result of premarital examinations are not routinely compiled. However, some special studies and surveys have been conducted which indicate that premarital testing remains productive. The results of a questionnaire sent to state health departments by the American Social Health Association indicate that premarital reactive rates for 28 states reporting were slightly higher than 1 percent in 1966.[8] A 1959 survey of premarital tests results in Georgia revealed that 1 percent of 25,000 persons tested needed treatment for syphilis.[9] Between 1949 and 1951, 4.3 percent of the primary and secondary syphilis cases reported in California were brought to treatment as a result of premarital examinations.[10]

Prenatal Examinations

A serologic test for syphilis for pregnant women before or after delivery is required in forty-two states.[11] Like the premarital examination, this procedure has been widely followed since World War II and is designed to reduce congenital syphilis among newborn children. In this respect these tests have been remarkably effective. Cases of congenital syphilis of less than one year's duration occur almost exclusively among infants born of women who receive little or no prenatal care and who deliver at home or first receive medical attention during delivery at a hospital. With the medical facilities available in the United States today, there is little excuse for the delivery of an infected infant.

The results of the same questionnaire sent to state health departments by the American Social Health Association indicate that reactivity rates among pregnant women were about 1 percent in 1966.[12]

Despite the marked decline in the past two decades of the total number of reported cases of congenital syphilis, recent figures show an increase of congenital syphilis among newborn children since 1957. The reported incidence of congenital syphilis under one year parallels the reported incidence of primary and secondary cases among females during the same period (Table 4.1). Such increases would seem to represent casefinding failure and inadequate prenatal medical care.

Table 4.1   Comparison of reported case rates of congenital syphilis cases under one year with reported case rates for primary and secondary syphilis for females: United States, fiscal years 1957-66

Fiscal year	Congenital syphilis under one year, cases per 10,000 live births	Primary and secondary syphilis for females, cases per 100,000 population
1957	0.4	2.6
1958	0.5	2.7
1959	0.5	2.9
1960	0.5	4.2
1961	0.8	6.5
1962	0.8	7.4
1963	0.9	8.4
1964	0.8	8.7
1965	0.8	9.1
1966	1.0	8.8

Examinations on Admission to Hospitals

Today only about one-half of the nation's hospitals perform routine serologic tests for syphilis on patients admitted for hospital care.[13] At one time such tests were routine in all accredited hospitals, but rising medical costs and minimal yields from the examinations caused the Joint Commission on Hospital Accreditation to delete serologic testing as an accreditation requirement in late 1955.[14] Because of the rise in the incidence of early syphilis, in 1965 the Association of State and Territorial Health Officers, the American Social Health Association, and the American Venereal Disease Association recommended the reinstatement of serological tests on all routine hospital admissions.[15]

In a national survey conducted in 1962, 6,424 hospitals reported that 3.1 percent of the approximately 17 million specimens were reactive.[16] As shown in Figure 4.1, the percentage of reactive specimens varied considerably by type of hospital. Reactivity ranged from a high of 7.0 percent for tuberculosis hospitals to a low of 1.6 percent for short-term and long-term proprietary hospitals. The 3.1 percent over-all reactivity in hospitals correlates with a 4.0 percent reactive rate as reported in a national probability sample of the adult population in 1962.[17]

Red Cross and Blood Bank Programs

Blood donor agencies perform serologic tests for syphilis on all specimens. As with other screening programs the yield has declined, both because syphilis is less prevalent and because blood donors are screened for history of infection before donating. Known syphilitics and persons whose general health is poor or questionable are usually excluded. Even if there is a false negative laboratory test in an infectious patient or if a patient has sero-negative primary syphilis, there is little danger of transmitting syphilis to the recipient if the blood is handled through the usual blood bank procedures. After seventy-two hours in a refrigerator (42° F) syphilitic blood is thought to be noninfectious. Though blood donor programs undoubtedly serve as an excellent surveillance device, their exact contribution to syphilis control is difficult to evaluate, because cases reported to the Public Health Service are not classified in specific detail as to the original reason for diagnosis.

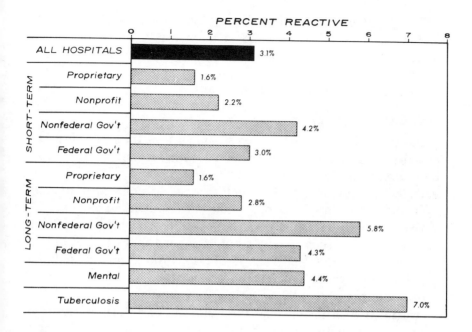

Fig. 4.1. Percent reactive specimens in serological tests for syphilis on routine hospital admissions, by type of hospital; national survey, 1962.

Source: W.J. Brown and J.A. Mahoney, "Serologic Tests for Syphilis: A Profile of Hospital Practice," *Journal of the American Hospital Association,* 37:66 (Nov. 1, 1963).

Pre-employment Examinations

In past years serologic tests for syphilis in pre-employment examinations were standard practice for thousands of industrial firms in the United States. Reactivity rates varied according to occupation.

In reviewing the literature, Stokes (1938) found that rates ran from as high as 11 percent among some unskilled groups to less than 1 percent among professionals. He quotes Lewis as saying that in agricultural and industrial labor in the South, rates ran as high as 12-35 percent.[18] In 1943 Anderson estimated that almost 1.3 million industrial workers were infected with syphilis.[19] As recently as 1954 a survey conducted among 15,000 persons in Washington, D.C., revealed an over-all reactivity rate of 9 percent, with about one in every three persons with reactive tests needing treatment.[20] These rates were high because of the selective nature of the survey.

Today pre-employment serologic examinations produce a lower number of cases than they did in past years. Although more and more industrial concerns require physical examinations, fewer require serologic tests. As a result, this source of surveillance activity will be of limited usefulness in the future.

Selectees and Separatees

Military physical examinations in all branches of the service include a serologic examination on incoming and outgoing members, a procedure which has been followed since World War I. These tests have detected thousands of cases and at one time provided our best estimates of the prevalence of syphilis in the United States.

The syphilis rate per 1,000 young adults examined for military service has declined markedly from 45.3 per 1,000 selectees in 1941 to 1.6 per 1,000 selectees in 1956. In 1966 approximately 400 syphilis cases were brought to treatment by health departments throughout the United States from selectee testing.

Overall, it is estimated that the follow-up of all reactive serologic tests brought to treatment about 29 percent of all newly reported primary and secondary syphilis cases, and 37 percent of all reported early latent syphilis cases in the United States in 1966.

SYPHILIS EPIDEMIOLOGY

Epidemiology is the science concerned with the factors and conditions that determine the occurrence and distribution of disease. In syphilis control the word epidemiology is used in a somewhat restricted sense, because the control procedures emphasize results in terms of treatment and prevention of spread rather than detailed and precise accounts of the circumstances surrounding each infection. As applied to syphilis control, epidemiology usually refers to tracing the source and spread of infections by interviewing known patients for sex contacts and cluster suspects and by investigating these contacts and cluster suspects to detect infections.

The epidemiologic approach to syphilis is limited in the sense that it controls infections but is not fully preventive. For its operation, at least one case must be acquired, diagnosed, and reported before remedial measures are introduced. However, until research in syphilis immunology produces a vaccine, epidemiology appears to be the best alternative solution yet developed for control. It is still the most important arm of the syphilis control program in the United States.

Signs and symptoms often do not alert infected patients sufficiently to seek diagnosis; therefore, rapid investigation of sex contacts is essential in bringing these persons to treatment. The importance of epidemiology is also substantiated by a nationwide study in 1963 in which 45 percent of persons brought to treatment as sex contacts admitted that they had recognized signs and/or symptoms but did not seek medical advice.

Epidemiology, when geared to a program of control and eradication, usually consists of four basic techniques:

1. Effectively interviewing and reinterviewing every reported early syphilis patient for sex contacts.

2. Rapid investigation to bring contacts to medical examination within a minimal time period.

3. Interviewing for and blood testing other persons who by definition (*suspect* or *associate*) are possibly involved sexually in an infectious chain (cluster procedure). This technique is designed to motivate the patients not only to name contacts but to name persons other than sex contacts for whom an examination for syphilis would seem profitable (cluster suspects). In addition, when named contacts are investigated, they are also asked to indicate persons in their social group whom they feel would likewise benefit from an examination (cluster associates). In the United States promiscuous persons behave sexually in somewhat similar patterns. Because of the continuous association within the same community groups, experience indicates that infectious patients and their contacts possess information concerning the sexual behavior of other group members. They also have knowledge of persons with signs or symptoms of syphilis. This information has been productive in bringing persons with syphilis to treatment.

4. Epidemiologic (preventive or prophylactic) treatment of sex contacts to infectious syphilis cases.

The interview of the infectious patient for contacts and suspects is the first step in the epidemiologic process. This interview must be performed so effectively that the information obtained will result in finding all contacts exposed within the period of infectivity and in finding any additional persons (suspects) of the same social-sexual groups that may have been exposed to an infectious person. To perform this interview, a worker must have a thorough knowledge of the medical and etiologic aspects of syphilis as well as training in methods of interviewing and finding people on the basis of minimal information.

Interviewing is simple in theory, but complex in practice. Its complexities result from the patient's attitude toward the interview itself, and indeed the barriers set up by the patient may, to him, be very justifiable. He may resent his diagnosis and the social overtones of the diagnosis. He is concerned about discussing his behavior with a stranger. He thinks loyalty to others is maintained by silence or giving incorrect information. He fears family or marital discord or a loss of community status. Many other reasons may decrease the success of an interview. The degree of success rests with how well the interviewer removes these barriers and elicits the information necessary to find the contacts or suspects in order to identify the probable source and bring to treatment the possible spread cases.

Of the 22,473 infectious syphilis cases reported in fiscal year 1966, 38 percent were brought to treatment through epidemiologic follow-up of known cases. The intensity of this type of casefinding strongly influences the reported incidence of primary and secondary syphilis. Table 4.2 illustrates the marked improvement which occurred during the last decade. The number of primary and secondary syphilis cases brought to treatment through epidemiology increased for ten consecutive years (1956-1965). This number decreased slightly during 1966 compared to 1965, a decrease that is in accord with the decrease noted in the total. From 1959 to 1963, an average of 34 percent of all primary and secondary syphilis cases were detected epidemiologically. For the period 1954 to 1958, an average of 19 percent were brought to treatment through epidemiologic follow-up. The marked increase in the percentage of infectious syphilis cases brought to treatment as a result of epidemiologic follow-up reflects the nationwide increase in intensive casefinding activity which has occurred since 1960. After severe federal budget cuts in 1954, state venereal disease control programs operated on a restricted basis. Few health departments were able to provide the necessary personnel to follow adequately reported cases of infectious syphilis. As a result, few cases were brought to treatment epidemiologically during the period 1954-1958.

It is likely that some of the cases which were not detected by health department workers were eventually diagnosed and treated by private physicians or clinics as a result of patients volunteering or through the follow-up of reactive serologic tests reported by laboratories. However, not all patients were treated, and many of those who received treatment had already progressed through infectious stages. This is illustrated in Table 4.3 by the high ratio of early latent

Table 4.2   Primary and secondary syphilis cases brought to treatment as a result of syphilis epidemiology: United States, fiscal years 1956-66

| Fiscal year | Primary and secondary syphilis cases | | |
| | Brought to treatment through epidemiology | | Total reported cases |
	Number	Percent	Number
1956	1,220	19.2	6,362 a
1957	1,377	22.0	6,251
1958	1,571	23.6	6,661
1959	2,318	28.5	8,124 b
1960	3,770	30.2	12,471
1961	6,706	35.7	18,772
1962	7,135	35.5	20,084
1963	7,599	34.5	22,045
1964	8,152	35.9	22,733
1965	9,002	38.7	23,250
1966	8,607	38.3	22,473

Sources: Public Health Service 9.688 Venereal Disease Morbidity Report and Public Health Service 9.2127 Quarterly Epidemiologic Activity Report.

a 47 states reporting.
b 48 states reporting.

Table 4.3   Cases of syphilis reported to the Public Health Service: United States, fiscal years 1954-63 (Known military cases are excluded)

Fiscal year	Primary and secondary	Early latent	Ratio of early latent cases to primary and secondary cases
1954	7,688	24,999	3.3 to 1.0
1955	6,516	21,553	3.3 to 1.0
1956	6,757	20,014	3.0 to 1.0
1957	6,251	19,046	3.0 to 1.0
1958	6,661	16,698	2.5 to 1.0
1959	8,178	17,592	2.2 to 1.0
1960	12,471	16,829	1.3 to 1.0
1961	18,781	19,146	1.0 to 1.0
1962	20,084	19,924	1.0 to 1.0
1963	22,045	18,683	0.8 to 1.0

cases to primary and secondary cases in the first period as compared to the second. When there is little or no casefinding activity it is probable that many infected persons will progress through the primary and secondary stages to latency before being detected. In fact, the continuing high number of reported cases of late and late latent syphilis indicate that some cases may lie hidden for years before finally being diagnosed and treated. This is harmful to the infected individual and dangerous for the public health control for it means that maximum spread occurred during primary, secondary, and in some instances, infectious relapse, stages.

During the period 1959 to 1963, epidemiologic efforts increased considerably, particularly after the Task Force Report on Syphilis was published early in 1962.[21] As a result of recommendations of this committee, the number of venereal disease field workers more than doubled. State programs developed and expanded. The increase in the number of cases detected epidemiologically is closely correlated with the increased number of personnel.

The increasing percentage of primary and secondary syphilis cases interviewed also reflects the increased number of personnel working in this area (Table 4.4). During 1966, 97.4 percent of primary and secondary syphilis cases were interviewed, as compared with 82.8 percent in 1960 and 90.5 percent in 1962, the first year after the Task Force Report was implemented. Most of the additional cases interviewed were cases reported by private physicians. In fiscal year 1966, 92.3 percent of the primary and secondary syphilis cases reported by private physicians were interviewed as compared to 61.7 percent in 1960.

To illustrate geographic variation in cases brought to treatment epidemiologically, Figure 4.2 analyzes the percentage of primary and secondary syphilis cases during the two five-year periods, 1954-1958 and 1959-1963. Probably most significant are the higher percentages of cases which were brought to treatment epidemiologically in southeastern states in the 1954-1958 period.

As the map for the 1959-1963 period indicates, the percentages of cases detected epidemiologically have climbed in most states outside the southeastern states. States with a high percentage of cases

Table 4.4   Percent of primary and secondary syphilis cases interviewed for contacts: United States, fiscal years 1960-66

Source	1960	1961	1962	1963	1964	1965	1966
All Sources	82.8	90.0	90.5	91.8	94.4	96.3	97.4
Public Cases	95.6	97.6	96.9	97.6	98.7	99.9	99.9
Private Cases	61.7	74.5	78.2	81.8	87.2	89.6	92.3

Sources: Public Health Service 9.688 Venereal Disease Morbidity Report and Public Health Service 9.2127 Quarterly Epidemiologic Activity Report.

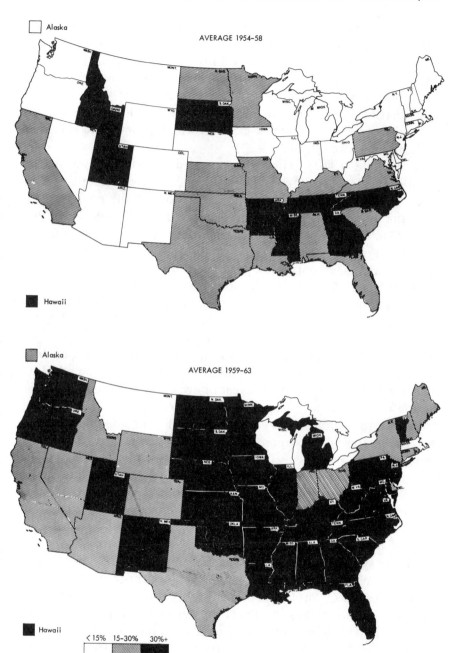

Fig. 4.2. Percent primary and secondary syphilis cases brought to treatment as a result of epidemiology: each state, averages for 1954-58 and 1959-63.

brought to treatment epidemiologically are usually states with high over-all case rates, while those with low brought-to-treatment percentages are those with low morbidity. Exceptions are New York, Illinois, and California where a high number of cases occur in the metropolitan areas, yet there is a low epidemiologic yield. This suggests that in order to obtain meaningful epidemiologic results, a substantial number of cases must exist on which an intensive epidemiologic program can operate.

In the late 1940's when the reported primary and secondary syphilis incidence was considerably higher, aggregate statistical indices were primarily used in the evaluation of the epidemiologic program. Four statistical measures of program efficiency were utilized. One is the contact index, which refers to the average number of critical period sex contacts obtained per case interviewed. A critical period sex contact is a person with whom the patient has had sexual contact while in an infectious stage. For primary syphilis, the critical period is 90 days (maximum incubation period) plus the length of time the patient has had his signs or symptoms. For the secondary stage, the critical period is six months (incubation plus primary period) plus the length of time secondary symptoms have been present. For early latent syphilis, the patient may be asked for all sex partners in the previous year or even four years, depending on the definition of early latency used. Obviously there may be some error due to faulty memory or the possibility of infectious relapse, but for interviewing purposes these critical periods have been satisfactory.

Contact indices will vary according to the skill of the interviewer and the type of patient. Most significant, however, is the nationwide increase from two contacts per patient interviewed in 1948 to four contacts per patient interviewed in 1964, indicating that good training and practical application of knowledge appears to be very productive in syphilis epidemiology (Figure 4.3).

The other indices are the epidemiologic, brought-to-treatment, and lesion-to-lesion. Of these, the brought-to-treatment index is probably the most important, for it reflects the detection of new cases in the population. This index is the total number of infected contacts of all stages brought to treatment per patient interviewed. Until it can be determined that the incidence of syphilis is decreasing, a higher number of cases brought to treatment through epidemiologic investigation is probably desirable, for it indicates that casefinding is

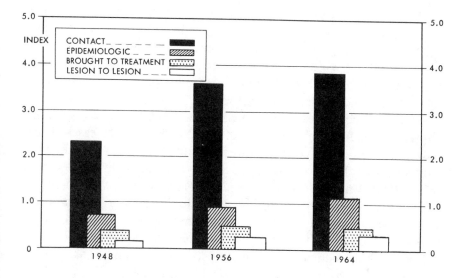

Fig. 4.3. Venereal disease epidemiologic indices, based on clinic primary and secondary syphilis patients: United States, 1948, 1956, and 1964.

effective. However, when syphilis incidence starts to decline, the number of cases detected through epidemiologic investigations may also decline.

While the brought-to-treatment index is concerned only with new cases, the epidemiologic index relates to previously treated contacts as well. The epidemiologic index is the total number of cases of syphilis identified among the contacts per patient interviewed. Since it includes previously treated contacts, the epidemiologic index will almost always be greater than and never less than the brought-to-treatment index. The epidemiologic index also contains late, congenital, and other early cases coincidentally detected in the process of investigation of contacts, but this number is minimal. The epidemiologic index is for practical purposes equal to the early cases brought to treatment plus the early cases previously treated.

The lesion-to-lesion index is a measure used to relate patients treated in a lesion stage (primary or secondary) with other lesion cases among contacts named by the patient. The lesion-to-lesion index is the total number of contacts diagnosed primary or secondary per primary or secondary patient interviewed. It is a measure of the speed and effectiveness of the epidemiological process, for, when investigations are rapidly initiated and completed, there is a greater likelihood that spread cases, and sometimes the source case, can be detected in a lesion stage. It is vital to do so, for early treatment prevents further spread. A high lesion-to-lesion index may indicate effective interviewing and rapid investigation. A low index may mean inadequate personnel to handle case loads as well as ineffective interviewing and contact investigation.

Figure 4.3 compares these four indices for selected years for the United States for clinic primary and secondary syphilis cases. There have been moderate, consistent increases in all indices other than the contact index. However, the application of epidemiologic treatment to contacts who are negative clinically and serologically in recent years is a significant factor in evaluating improvements in these casefinding indices since many spread cases are prevented. In areas where epidemiologic treatment is practiced, low lesion-to-lesion and brought-to-treatment indices are almost inevitable and consequently are not fair measurements of program effectiveness.

Epidemiologic or preventive treatment is the treatment of contacts exposed to primary or secondary syphilis who are negative clinically and serologically on initial examination. In a preventive therapy evaluation trial, 10 percent of the negative contacts exposed to primary or secondary syphilis who were given a placebo injection instead of one of the study drugs developed syphilis during the three month follow-up period.[22] With widespread use of epidemiologic treatment, the identification of the source contact and the failure to identify the source or any probable spread of infection appear to be relevant measurements of evaluation. In fiscal year 1966 states that completed source-spread reports found the probable source contact for 63.4 percent of the primary and secondary syphilis cases interviewed (Table 4.5). For interviewed cases, the probable source was found for 64.6 percent of the primary cases and 62.4 percent of the secondary cases.

A significant difference was noted between primary and secondary cases in determining spread of infection, although there is only a slight difference in locating the source contact. Spread cases were identified for 38.6 percent of secondary cases interviewed as compared to 18.2 percent of primary cases interviewed. Approximately one of every three primary cases and one of every four secondary cases result in a failure to identify a source or spread of infection. This appears to be high, but represents a considerable improvement. Over-all, 26.6 percent of the primary and secondary cases interviewed in 1966 were classified as a failure to identify source or

Table 4.5   Source and spread results for primary and secondary syphilis cases
interviewed: 47 project states reporting, fiscal years 1964 and 1966

Diagnosis; year	Cases interviewed Number	Source contact		One or more spread contacts		No source or spread contacts	
		Number	Percent	Number	Percent	Number	Percent
Total							
1964	21,354	12,984	60.8	6,243	29.2	6,179	28.9
1966	21,855	13,854	63.4	6,346	29.0	5,804	26.6
Primary							
1964	9,793	6,135	62.6	1,936	19.8	3,166	32.3
1966	10,233	6,607	64.6	1,864	18.2	3,183	31.3
Secondary							
1964	11,561	6,849	59.2	4,307	37.3	3,013	26.1
1966	11,622	7,247	62.4	4,482	38.6	2,621	22.6

Sources: Public Health Service 9.70 Monthly Evaluation of Epidemiology of
Primary and Secondary Syphilis Cases and Public Health Service 9.77 Individual Case
Evaluation of Infectious Syphilis Epidemiology.

spread as compared to 37.4 percent in 1960, the first year this type
of epidemiologic information was collected routinely. Most of the
improvement appears to be related to the increase in the number of
workers, which enabled each worker to put more intensive effort
into each case, and an over-all improvement in the application of
interviewing and investigating techniques.

With the improvements noted in syphilis epidemiology involving
sex contacts, a significant number of socially-related persons also
have been brought to treatment through cluster casefinding techniques since the late 1950's. The first attempts to apply cluster
techniques emphasized geographic blood testing involving reported
primary or secondary syphilis cases, particularly in rural areas.

In 1963 a pilot study of 1,256 primary and secondary syphilis
cases was conducted in eight states to determine the effectiveness of
intensified interviewing of infectious syphilis patients and their sex
contacts for other socially and sexually related persons that might
need an examination for syphilis. The study involved two major
groups: cluster suspects named by the infectious patient and cluster
associates named by sex contacts of the patient.

Cluster suspects named by the infectious patient were put in three
groups. The first group consisted of persons that the patient thought
had clinical signs or symptoms similar to his own. The study indicated that about one in eleven of such named persons will be brought

to treatment for syphilis. The yield from this type of suspect approximated the yield from contacts to primary and secondary syphilis cases. The second group of suspects consisted of persons the patient thought were sex partners or very close friends of other persons known by health authorities to be infected. One of every twenty-three of such suspects was brought to treatment for syphilis. The yield compares favorably to sex contacts for early latent syphilis cases. The last group of suspects consisted of members of the patient's household or family not designated as sex contacts by the patient. One of every thirty-three of these suspects was brought to treatment for syphilis.

The other category consisted of persons named by the sex contacts themselves. In this study, when sex contacts were persuaded to talk about other members of their group having clinical signs or symptoms suggestive of syphilis, one of every thirty named by these contacts required treatment. Many of the contacts interviewed suggested persons who were having sexual relations with other known cases in their group; one of every thirty-five required treatment for syphilis. Geographic blood testing resulted in very low yields in bringing persons to treatment with syphilis.

The study showed that in addition to an untreated case of syphilis being brought to treatment as a sex contact in one of every two cases interviewed, an untreated case was also brought-to-treatment as a socially related group suspect or associate in one of every seven primary or secondary cases interviewed. The study indicated that interviewing appears to be effective in developing a cluster with a satisfactory casefinding yield. Today the cluster technique is employed extensively throughout the United States together with contact epidemiology.

In summary, the modern syphilis control program in the United States communicates to the general public, specifically young adults and teenagers, the medical facts about syphilis to motivate them to voluntarily seek treatment if there are clinical or exposure indications. It applies epidemiologic techniques effectively to early syphilis cases through interviewing, investigation, and the cluster procedure. It provides preventive therapy for persons exposed to syphilis in an infectious stage who are negative clinically and serologically on first examination. It continues existing routine blood testing surveillance programs and employs mass or selective blood testing when indicated.

Although gonorrhea remains a major public health problem in the United States, the lack of a quick and accurate diagnostic method for the female has discouraged any organized control program since the middle 1950's.

5 / Morbidity

Definitions

Syphilis morbidity is generally defined as the aggregate of all cases reported for a specific population group for a specified period of time. Morbidity is influenced by prevalence and incidence, and these in turn influence one another. High prevalence is likely to reflect high incidence, and high incidence will contribute to prevalence by creating a reservoir of undetected or untreated cases.

The prevalence of syphilis is simply the total number of cases of the disease needing treatment at a particular point in time. Incidence, on the other hand, may be described in three ways: (1) *true incidence*, the number of cases actually occurring in a particular area during a specified period of time; (2) *diagnosed incidence*, the number of cases coming to medical attention; and (3) *reported incidence*, the number of diagnosed cases reported to the health department (or, on a national scale, to the Public Health Service). Of these, actual incidence is greatest, for it is unlikely that 100 percent of all persons infected with syphilis will seek or receive medical care. In addition, diagnosed incidence is usually greater than reported incidence, for many cases are, for one reason or another, not made known to health departments. Although the prevalence and incidence of syphilis cannot be determined by directly referring to reported figures, estimates of these measures can be made.

Prevalence of Venereal Disease

From the records of serologic and physical examinations of inductees at the time of their entry on active duty, the United States military services have compiled figures which, in the past, have been used to estimate the prevalence of venereal disease in the entire United States population. A study of the physical examinations of servicemen during World War I indicated that at the time of induction, 5.6 percent of a total of 3,500,000 men were infected with some type of venereal disease.[1] Another 2 percent acquired infection while on active duty, so that by the end of the war, approximately 7.5 percent of men between the ages of 18 and 35 were venereally infected. From these figures some authorities estimated that possibly 10 percent of the United States population was infected with at least one of the venereal diseases at the time of World War I.

By World War II, the value of serologic tests was well established, and the results of these tests were listed separately on the records of all inductees. Of the first two million men tested, 4.5 percent had reactive tests for syphilis. On the basis of these tests, the Public Health Service estimated that about 3,303,000 or 2.5 percent of the total United States population was infected with some stage of syphilis at the beginning of World War II. Since results from World War I examinations include all venereal diseases while those for World War II include only syphilis, the two figures are not directly comparable.

The Prevalence of Syphilis Today

From 1960 to 1962 the Public Health Service conducted a multi-phasic Health Examination Survey on a sample of 7,000 persons located in the continental United States. The several tests and examinations made during this survey were designed to measure the extent of selected health problems in the total population. One of the examinations given was a serologic test for syphilis,[2] and from the results an estimate of the prevalence of the disease can be made. Projected reactivity rates from the sample of 7,000 persons aged 18-79 years indicated that in the total non-institutionalized adult population of 140,000,000 at age 14 and over, approximately 4,000,000 had reactive serologic tests. This figure, however, did not represent the prevalence of syphilis, for it included a relatively small number of uninfected persons who had biologic false positive (BFP) reactions and excluded a small number of infected persons who were serologically negative (very early or very late cases). Most important, many of the 4,000,000 reactors were persons who had been adequately treated in the past but whose blood still remained reactive. Since these people were not part of the untreated syphilis reservoir, they must be excluded if a reasonable estimate of prevalence is to be achieved. This can be done by examining the results of reactor follow-up data tabulated by the national syphilis control program.

In many states, reactive tests are reported to local or state health departments. Between 1962 and 1965 about 20 percent of reported reactors were diagnosed as either previously untreated or inadequately treated. If, then, the estimated 4,000,000 reactors were tested and available at one time, about 20 percent or 800,000 could be expected to need treatment for some stage of syphilis. This figure represents an estimate of the prevalence of syphilis in the United States as of 1965.

Incidence

Incidence is a second component of morbidity which has significant implications for the syphilis control program. Since reported figures do not reflect the extent of occurrence, true incidence, like true prevalence, must be estimated. This would be no problem if all diagnosed cases were reported. Unfortunately, underreporting by private physicians is one of the major obstacles to the current control program, hampering epidemiologic control efforts and interfering with accurate assessment of the problem itself. In 1963 some indication of the extent of underreporting became available when the results of a study by the American Social Health Association became known.[3] The ASHA mailed a letter and a brief questionnaire to each of the 183,000 physicians in private practice in the United States asking for his confidential reply to three questions:

1. How many cases of infectious syphilis did you treat in the period April 1 – June 30, 1962?
2. How many cases of other stages of syphilis?
3. How many cases of gonorrhea?

The results for the fiscal year 1962, based upon returns from the 131,245 physicians who replied, are as follows:

	Reported number of cases	Estimated actual number of cases
Infectious syphilis	20,084	68,977
Other stages of syphilis	104,104	190,370
Gonorrhea	260,468	817,713

The estimated actual number of cases included those treated but unreported, as well as all cases reported.

The results of this survey correlate roughly with the findings of a study done by Lentz in Philadelphia in 1952, in which he found that about 25 percent of the syphilis cases treated by private physicians in that year had actually been reported.[4]

The results of the American Social Health Association study (1962) indicated that approximately 70,000 primary and secondary syphilis cases were being diagnosed and treated annually in the United States. During 1962 only about 20,000 primary and secondary syphilis cases were reported to health officials. Thus, it is evident that only a fraction of the diagnosed and treated cases of primary and secondary syphilis are being reported to health officials, and this hampers effective syphilis control since epidemiology cannot be carried out to determine the source and possible spread infections until a case is reported.

Nationwide data collected by the Venereal Disease Program on the results of reactor follow-up in conjunction with the National Health Survey data indicate that about 2 percent or 80,000 of the estimated 4,000,000 persons in the United States with a reactive test for syphilis acquired the disease (estimated incidence) during 1965.

The rising trend in the number of early cases reported between 1957 and 1965 indicates that penicillin alone is not enough to eradicate the disease. Until a greater number of cases are treated in the infectious stage of the disease, the reporting gap closed, and epidemiology applied to more cases, syphilis eradication will undoubtedly remain an objective rather than a reality.

Private Physician Cases

During the period between World War I and World War II, several surveys were conducted by the Venereal Disease Division to determine the number of persons under treatment for syphilis and gonorrhea. These "One-Day Surveys," as they were called, were conducted to provide an estimate of the extent of venereal disease in the population. At the time of the surveys, patients being treated for syphilis and gonorrhea were under long-term therapy; consequently, the magnitude of the venereal disease problem could be assessed by determining the number of patients individual physicians had under treatment as of a given day. From this procedure, the "One-Day Surveys" acquired their name.

Questionnaires were sent by mail; nonrespondents received a second questionnaire, telephone call, or visit from a health department representative. In this way an average response of about 90 percent was obtained. Both private physicians and those practicing in health department clinics were included in the sample. They were asked to provide two figures: the number of cases of syphilis and the number of cases of gonorrhea under treatment on the day of the survey. The findings were then tabulated and analyzed.

Table 5.1 provides a summary of the results of a number of selected surveys. These figures were derived from reports appearing in issues of the *Journal of Venereal Disease Information* and in other medical journals between 1926 and 1931. The communities listed do not include all of those which were ever surveyed, but represent a cross-section of several areas in the United States. Results indicate that an average of two-thirds (67 percent) of all cases under treatment on the several different survey days were treated by private physicians. Many, particularly those in large cities, were treated by a

Table 5.1   Cases of syphilis and gonorrhea under observation or treatment[a]: results from one-day surveys conducted from 1926 to 1930

Community	Total number of responding physicians	Physicians treating one or more cases of syphilis and/or gonorrhea		Cases under treatment or observation in private practice		Cases under treatment or observation in public clinics	
		Number	Percent	Number	Percent	Number	Percent
Peoria, Ill.	169		53		85		15
Huntington, W. Va.	102		48		75		25
Wheeling, W. Va.	80		63		71		29
Decatur, Ill.	77		51		62		38
Lexington, Ky.	105		49		44		56
El Dorado, Ark.	36		50		100		
Paducah, Ky.	44	454	52	5,395	94	1,789	6
Texarkana, Ark.	45		67		100		-
LaSalle District, Ill.[b]	25		60		100		-
Pike County, Ky.	29		60		100		-
Logan County, W. Va.	42		69		77		23
Morgan County, Ill.	40		53		96		4
Greenbrier C., W. Va.	21		38		100		-
Scott Co., Ky.	18		50		51		49
Detroit, Mich.	1,773	851	48	11,629	69	5,106	31
Cleveland, Ohio	1,475	671	45	7,558	58	5,452	42
Upstate N. Y.[c]	5,340	2,230	42	19,516	74	6,954	26
22 Kansas Counties[d]	742	314	42	3,135	96	114	4
Oregon	1,233	489	40	4,333	89	546	11
34 Tennessee Cos.	1,590	728	46	7,803	69	3,543	31
16 Mississippi Cos.	484	277	57	3,714	88	488	12
St. Louis, Mo.	2,096	1,037	49	11,778	78	3,324	22
18 Virginia Cos.	1,101	566	51	6,694	79	1,781	21
Philadelphia, Pa.	3,351	1,042	31	8,425	45	10,384	55
Brooklyn, N. Y.	2,625	997	38	8,595	80	2,101	20
Baltimore, Md.	1,120	271	24	3,003	28	7,704	72
Charleston, W. Va.	114	55	48	1,031	60	677	40
All Communities	23,877	9,982	42	102,609	67	49,963	33

Source: Various issues of the Journal of Venereal Disease Information and other medical journals between 1926 and 1931.
    a. See text for discussion of data.
    b. Includes LaSalle, Oglesby, and Peru.
    c. Excludes New York City.
    d. Clinics in two counties only.

few specialists; nevertheless, 42 percent of all responding physicians were treating one or more cases of venereal disease. The proportion of cases being treated by private physicians ranged from as low as 28 percent in Baltimore to as high as 100 percent in some small rural communities. In general, the larger the city the greater the likelihood that a larger percentage of cases were treated in clinics. In smaller towns and rural areas, the percentage of cases treated in clinics was probably lower because clinic facilities were often not available. In most instances private physicians treated more cases of gonorrhea than syphilis, but syphilis cases still constituted a sizeable segment of their venereal disease practice. In Virginia, for example, 49 percent of all cases under treatment on the day of the survey were syphilis cases.

The exigencies of World War II undoubtedly caused a shift of patients from private treatment facilities to public treatment facilities. The short intensive schedules for syphilis therapy could be given only on an inpatient basis, and beginning in 1942, health department Rapid Treatment Centers were established throughout the nation to treat syphilis on an inpatient basis. Military selectees with syphilis were treated at these facilities before entering service. Rapid Treatment Centers also minimized work time lost among the civilian segment of the population. In 1944 penicillin for the treatment of syphilis was available only to these Rapid Treatment Centers. Not until 1947 or 1948 was the supply of penicillin sufficient to meet all of the needs of private medicine, nor were well evaluated and satisfactory schedules of syphilis therapy available for use on an outpatient basis.

Persons who worked in venereal disease control during World War II were firmly convinced that private physicians reported more of their cases during and shortly following the war than before or since. An accurate statistical picture of this improved wartime reporting is not available, but cases of primary and secondary syphilis reported by private physicians in the United States rose from 42.7 percent of all cases reported in fiscal year 1941 to 50.7 percent of all cases in 1942, despite a rise in public diagnostic activity due to Selective Service examining procedures.

The 1962 American Social Health Association survey suggests that possibly only 10-15 percent of all primary and secondary syphilis cases diagnosed by private physicians are reported. The results of this study also indicate that about 75-80 percent of all cases (public and private) diagnosed annually in the United States are diagnosed and treated by private physicians.[5]

The available data appear to indicate that even in the days when treatment was long, dangerous, and of uncertain value, the majority of cases under treatment were treated by private physicians. About the same proportion of cases are being treated by private physicians today as in the 1920's and 1930's.

The great decline in reported cases of early syphilis after 1947 is attributed by most authorities to an actual decline in disease incidence due to the greater proportion of cases available to health departments for epidemiologic studies during and shortly following World War II, coupled with a more efficacious treatment for syphilis, namely penicillin. A few attribute the decline in reported cases after 1947 to a shift of patients from public to private treatment facilities. The postwar decline of early syphilis cases is probably due to a combination of both of these factors – declining incidence and poorer case reporting.

Reported Cases of Syphilis

The Public Health Service issues uniform specifications for reporting venereal disease morbidity based on the recommendations of the Conference of State and Territorial Epidemiologists. For syphilis, reporting instructions specify that any case not previously reported in a state should be counted in the statistical summary of cases submitted periodically to the Public Health Service. Because syphilis, especially in the late and late latent stages, is manifested by reactive blood which may persist for many years, cases are subject to multiple diagnoses and case reports. In order to eliminate duplicate reports on the same patient, most state health departments maintain a central case register of all previously reported cases against which new case reports are matched before being included in the statistical summary of disease. However, according to the existing reporting rules, a case can be reported more than once if it is diagnosed and reported in more than one state. The extent of overreporting due to interstate mobility of syphilis patients is not known.

For early syphilis, duplicate case reporting is not a problem because adequate treatment quickly cures the disease and the blood soon returns to negative, thus minimizing the chances for a subsequent diagnosis and duplicate case report on the same patient in the same or a different state for the same infection.

Gonorrhea in the male is an acute condition quickly cured by adequate treatment. Multiple attacks of gonorrhea are considered to be reinfections and appear in the statistics as many times as patients acquire the disease. By and large, then, morbidity statistics for syphilis represent different persons with disease, whereas gonorrhea statistics reflect a count of infections, many of which occur in the same patient more than once.

Public Health Service morbidity statistics from most of the states for all stages of syphilis combined and for gonorrhea go back to the year 1919. Beginning in fiscal year 1941, all states began reporting syphilis by stage of disease, color, sex, and reporting source (private physicians or public clinics). Since 1956, primary and secondary syphilis and gonorrhea cases have been reported by age.

Disease Trends

Syphilis, All Stages

Figure 5.1 shows reported civilian cases of syphilis and gonorrhea per 100,000 population in the United States for each of the fiscal years 1919-1966. At least forty-one states and the District of Columbia reported cases in each of the years 1919 through 1938; after 1938 all states are included in the reporting area.

During the period 1919 through 1935, reported syphilis case rates gradually increased, rising from 113.2 cases per 100,000 population in 1919 to 212.6 cases per 100,000 population in 1936. During the same years, gonorrhea rates remained essentially level. It is doubtful if the doubling of reported syphilis rates was due so much to an increase in incidence and prevalence during these years as to a gradually increasing recognition of syphilis as a public health problem resulting in an increased level of casefinding and better case reporting.

During the middle 1930's public and governmental awareness of the venereal disease problem gathered momentum. The increasing publicity given to the venereal disease problem is illustrated by the fact that from 1932 to 1935, there were only 5 articles in the *New York Times* relating to venereal disease; during the next five years the *Times* carried 255 articles relating to venereal disease. Similar increases were noted in the number of venereal disease articles appearing in magazines.[6] Appropriations for venereal disease control

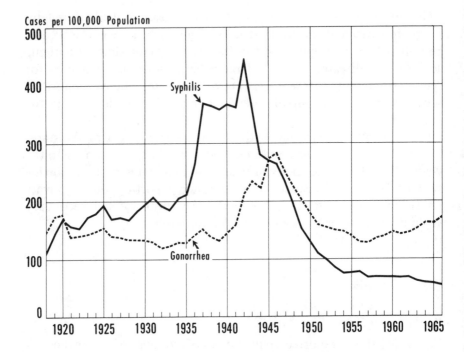

Fig. 5.1. Reported civilian case rates for syphilis and gonorrhea:* United States, fiscal years ending June 30, 1918 to 1966.

*Beginning with 1939, all states are included in the reporting area. Military cases are included from 1919 to 1940, but excluded thereafter.

increased from $80,000 in 1936 to $3,000,000 in 1938 and to over $4,500,000 in 1940. These federal appropriations were used to coordinate and supplement the control activities of state and local health services, which until this time had borne almost the entire fiscal burden of control activities.

The large increase in the reported case rate of syphilis which began in 1938 can be attributed to the nationwide intensification of case-finding activities. Casefinding was further intensified during World War II with the bloodtesting of nearly all young American males in connection with the physical examination for military service.

After World War II, casefinding activities were stepped up again among the civilian population by means of mass and selective blood-testing surveys in the urban and rural areas of much of the nation. Bloodtesting stations were set up in schools and churches, at the country crossroads, on street corners, and in bars. In some high prevalence areas, survey personnel carried their needles from door to door to insure maximum response to the survey appeal. This massive campaign was successful to the extent that by the mid-1950's most existing cases in the population had been detected. Accordingly, selective bloodtesting surveys were for the most part discontinued in the United States because of their lack of productivity in detecting previously unknown and untreated cases of syphilis.

The decrease in the reported syphilis case rate after 1943 can be attributed to two factors. The first of these is a decrease in the amount of casefinding activity. The most important reason, however, is the success of earlier casefinding efforts. The majority of syphilitics in the population had been previously detected, treated, and reported, and thus were not eligible for inclusion in the morbidity statistics. In the year ending June 30, 1965, casefinding workers followed to medical diagnosis 144,085 persons known to have a reactive test for syphilis. Only 25,070 of these 144,085 persons (17.4 percent) were diagnosed as having previously untreated syphilis.

Latent syphilis casefinding now depends on the massive network of compulsory and voluntary screening tests mentioned in the preceding chapter. Altogether, it is estimated that about 38,000,000 serologic tests for syphilis are performed each year or about one test for each five adults in the population. [7]

Primary and Secondary Syphilis Trends

Primary and secondary syphilis are the symptomatic infectious stages of recently acquired syphilis. The trend of reported cases of primary and secondary syphilis is interpreted as an index of the trend of actual occurrence of disease, because in these cases the disease has been recently acquired.

Reported infectious cases are not only a function of the number of cases occurring but are also a function of the proportion of cases which are diagnosed and the proportion of diagnosed cases which are reported. Therefore, changes in levels of casefinding and changes in case reporting practices can influence the trend of reported cases.

If physicians reported more, or less, of the cases they diagnosed, or if patients turned from private to public clinic diagnostic facilities, or vice versa, a different trend for private and for public cases of syphilis would be evident (see Table 5.2). However, changes in early syphilis casefinding activities or in reporting practices could not have accounted for the 40-50 percent per annum decreases and increases in reported cases which have occurred during the past twenty-five

Table 5.2   Cases of primary and secondary syphilis
             reported by private and public diagnostic
             facilities: United States, fiscal years
             1947, 1957, and 1966

| Fiscal year | Total, All Sources | Reporting Source | |
		Private	Public
1947	106,539	32,551	73,988
1957	6,251	2,573	3,678
1966	22,473	8,740	13,733

Source: PHS 9.688 Venereal Disease Morbidity Report,
submitted by states to the Public Health Service.

years. Therefore, reported cases of primary and secondary syphilis are interpreted as essentially paralleling the actual occurrence of disease, especially when the changes are sudden and large.

Figure 5.2 shows the trend of reported civilian cases of primary and secondary syphilis in the United States from fiscal years 1941 through 1966. In 1941, the first year in which all states reported infectious syphilis cases to the Public Health Service, state health departments reported a total of 68,231 cases. Reported cases increased yearly thereafter, with the exception of 1944 and 1945 when there were minor decreases, to an all-time high of 106,539 cases reported in 1947. Thereafter, the number of infectious cases decreased rapidly to 6,516 cases reported in 1955 -- the decrease amounting to as much as 40 percent per year during these eight years. Reported cases remained at about the 6,500 level through 1958, after which increases were noted again. These increases measured in the magnitude of 50 percent per year during 1960 and 1961. Since 1961 the rate of increase has not been as great, but the 23,250 cases reported in 1965 were almost four times the 6,251 cases reported in 1957, the all-time low year for reported cases of primary and secondary syphilis. In 1966 the number of such cases decreased slightly.

Early Latent Syphilis Trends

The trend of reported cases of early latent syphilis is shown in Fig. 5.2. Latent syphilis is the stage of the disease which follows the lesions and symptoms of the primary or secondary stage. The majority of states define the early latent stage as syphilis of less than four years' duration; a few states define it as syphilis of less than two

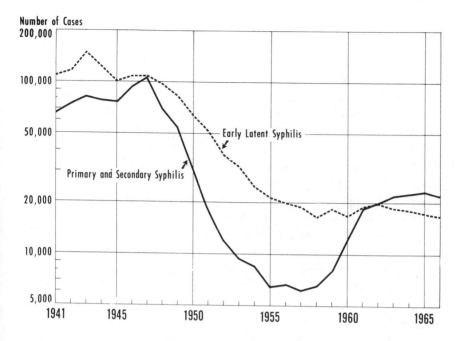

Fig. 5.2. Reported civilian case rates for syphilis by diagnosis: United States, fiscal years ending June 30, 1941 to 1966.

years' duration. Beginning about 1962, some state health departments changed the definition of early latent from syphilis of less than four years' duration to syphilis known to be of less than one year's duration. This change in definition may have had some effect on the trend of reported cases between 1962 and 1966, by causing fewer cases to be classified as early latent.

Because early latent syphilis is symptomless, the motivation to seek treatment afforded the primary and secondary syphilis patient by the presence of lesions is missing, and almost complete reliance has to be placed on serologic testing to detect early latent syphilis. Therefore, changes in the amount of bloodtesting in the population as well as changes in the attitudes of the private practitioner of medicine about case reporting can influence the trend of reported cases. But attitudes and casefinding activities are believed to change relatively slowly, and the trend of reported cases of early latent syphilis is interpreted as being a crude indicator of the actual trend of the prevalence of syphilis in its earliest period of latency.

The trend of reported cases of early latent syphilis (Figure 5.2) very roughly parallels the line for primary and secondary cases, decreasing from 107,767 cases reported in 1947 to 21,553 cases reported in 1955, a decrease of 80 percent compared to a decrease of 94 percent in primary and secondary cases over the same period of time. From 1961 through 1965, reported early latent syphilis cases decreased 10 percent while cases in the primary and secondary stage increased 24 percent.

There are several reasons why the trend of early latent cases is not more closely correlated with the trend of primary and secondary cases. First, primary and secondary cases are an immediate result of current disease incidence, whereas early latent cases are a result of incidence for the preceding two to four years. Therefore, early latent syphilis would reflect increases or decreases in incidence more slowly than primary and secondary syphilis, lagging behind perhaps as much as four years. Second, the precise determination of duration of disease (less than four or more than four years) is often difficult to make. In the absence of a history of infectious lesions, a negative bloodtest less than four years preceding diagnosis, or a history of exposure to an infectious case, the clinician must make an educated guess of the duration of disease in a latent syphilitic. In practice the age of the patient, in the absence of information to precisely pin-point the duration of disease, then becomes the deciding factor in classifying the disease as being of more or less than four (in some areas two) years' duration. Usually, in such cases those under twenty-six years of age are classed as early latent syphilis and those twenty-six years of age and over are classed as latent syphilis of more than four years' duration. To the extent that classification errors are made, the sensitivity of reported cases of early latent syphilis to reflect recent incidence is destroyed.

The ratio of the number of cases in the primary and secondary stage of syphilis to the number in the early latent stage and the changes in this ratio over the years have important control program implications. When this ratio is increasing, a greater proportion of the cases occurring are being detected in the infectious stage of disease and a smaller proportion are progressing into latency. The current syphilis control program is based on the premise that if a sufficient proportion of newly acquired cases can be detected while in the infectious stage and rendered noninfectious by means of treatment, then the spread of syphilis can be sufficiently reduced so that the results will be a continuous downward trend in syphilis incidence.

Reported early latent morbidity exceeded primary and secondary morbidity in every year from 1941 through 1961. Since 1961 there has been a steadily increasing excess of reported infectious syphilis cases over reported early latent syphilis cases in the United States.

Late and Late Latent Syphilis

The following abbreviated data (see also Tables A.I.1 and A.I.2) show the long-term trend of reported cases of late and late latent syphilis in the United States:

Fiscal year	Cases of syphilis	
	Late and late latent	All stages of syphilis
1943	251,958	575,593
1950	112,424	229,723
1955	84,741	122,075
1960	84,156	120,249
1966	66,149	110,128

Roughly one-half of all reported cases of syphilis are reported in the late and late latent stages of disease. Therefore, the trend of syphilis in all stages, discussed earlier, is largely dependent upon the trend of late and late latent syphilis. The Public Health Service does not have data which distinguish the frequency of late latent and of late syphilis.

In 1958 Canada reported that 6.7 percent of 1,692 reported cases of late and late latent syphilis were diagnosed as cardiovascular syphilis and an additional 13.4 percent were reported as neuro-syphilis. By 1964 the proportion of reported cases of late and late latent syphilis which were diagnosed as cardiovascular or neuro-syphilis had dropped to about one-half of the 1958 proportion.[8]

Since by definition the late latent stage of syphilis is clinically symptomless, there is little, if any, motivation of the infected individual to seek medical attention. Therefore, casefinding of latent syphilis is almost entirely by serologic testing--those tests required by law as well as tests optionally ordered by doctors, hospitals, and employers.

Finding and treating cases of syphilis in the latent stage prevents the development of the late debilitating manifestations. Since cases of late syphilis are not reported separately to the Public Health Service, data relating to admissions to mental hospitals with psychoses due to syphilis and mortality due to syphilis, discussed in Chapter 7, may be used to evaluate the impact of program efforts on the trends of late syphilis.

Congenital Syphilis

Reported cases of congenital syphilis numbered 17,600 cases in fiscal year 1941; 12,836 in 1951; 4,388 in 1961; and 3,464 in 1966.

Since most of reported cases are adults and these reported cases represent failure to prevent disease twenty or more years prior to detection, there is a lengthy time lag between institution of preventive measures and the reflection of the effectiveness of these measures in reported morbidity.

Congenital syphilis is almost completely preventable and institution of an effective preventive program would be reflected almost immediately by a decrease of syphilis in the newborn. Unfortunately, the Public Health Service does not have the data related to syphilis in the newborn for making comparisons before and after the implementation of the prenatal testing programs which were started in the late 1930's and early 1940's. The available Public Health Service information on reported congenital syphilis cases by age from fiscal year 1951 through fiscal year 1966 is listed in Table A.I.16. To adjust for the varying numbers of states which did not report cases by age during this time period, the distribution of cases with known age was extended to cases whose age was not reported to estimate the number of congenital syphilis cases under one year of age in the United States.

These data show a correlation between the reported incidence of congenital syphilis in infants and the incidence of syphilis in adults as measured by reported cases of syphilis in the primary and secondary stages of the disease. The estimated number of syphilis cases among infants decreased from 796 in 1951 to a low of 180 in 1957. The number of such cases then increased to a high of 410 noted in 1963 and dropped to about 370 cases annually for the next three years.

Geographic Distribution of Syphilis

Primary and Secondary Syphilis

Figure 5.3 shows the geographic distribution of rates of primary and secondary syphilis in fiscal year 1947, the year of highest reported

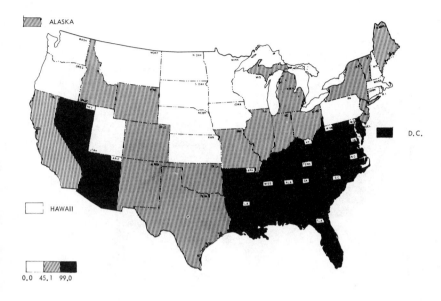

Fig. 5.3. Primary and secondary syphilis case rates per 100,000 population: each state, fiscal year ending June 30, 1947.

incidence of syphilis in the United States. In 1947 the rates ranged from a low of 16.5 cases per 100,000 population in Hawaii to a high of 360.9 in Mississippi. The high rate states were located predominantly in the Southeastern United States, and the intermediate rate states were generally contiguous to the high rate states. The low rate states were in the north central states, plus Oregon and Washington. Figure 5.4 shows the distribution of primary and secondary rates in fiscal year 1965. Infectious syphilis rates ranged from a low of 0.2 cases per 100,000 population in Vermont (only one case was reported) to a high of 69.4 cases per 100,000 population in the District of Columbia.

Comparison of Figures 5.3 and 5.4 indicates a somewhat greater dispersion of high incidence states in 1965 than in 1947, the movement of high incidence areas generally moving from South to North. Some of the formerly high rate states of the South, especially the border states, moved from the high rate to the intermediate rate classification while some of the northern industrial states (New York, New Jersey, Delaware, Maryland, and Illinois) moved from the intermediate rate classification into the category of high rate states.

Although there have been some changes over the years in the relative distribution of disease incidence, all states and cities have

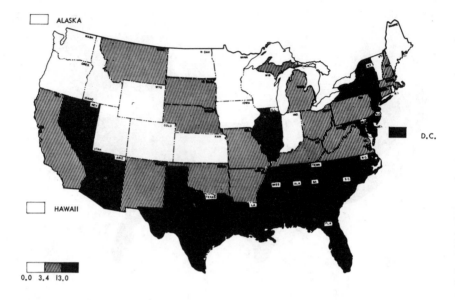

Fig. 5.4. Primary and secondary syphilis case rates per 100,000 population: each state, fiscal year ending June 30, 1965.

been remarkably consistent in following the ups and downs of reported syphilis incidence as indicated by the trend of the United States annual totals of primary and secondary cases. Trend data for each state and for major cities are presented in Tables A.I.4-14.

The racial composition of the population of any state is a very decided factor in its reported venereal disease rate. Since 1947 the changes in the geographic distribution of venereal disease incidence have been generally consistent with the differential migration patterns of whites and Negroes in the United States.

When adjustments are made for the disparate distribution of the white and nonwhite population among the states, much of the geographic pattern of disease incidence disappears. Figure 5.5 shows the geographic distribution of color adjusted rates of primary and secondary syphilis. These rates were computed by averaging the cases for fiscal years 1959, 1960, and 1961, computing color specific rates for each state, and using the 1950 United States census color composition as the standard population.

Late and Late Latent Syphilis

Reported case rates of late and late latent syphilis are extremely difficult to interpret for local areas in the absence of a considerable

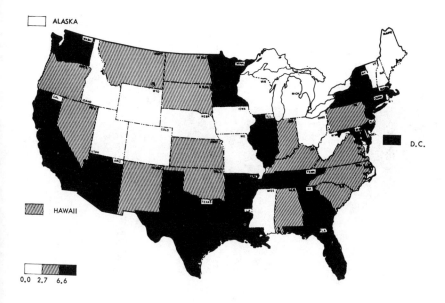

Fig. 5.5. Primary and secondary syphilis case rates per 100,000 population, race adjusted: each state, fiscal years ending June 30, 1959 to 1961.

knowledge about past and present health department operations, intensity of casefinding, migration patterns of syphilitics, and completeness of reporting. All of these factors can affect the reported case rate and affect its accuracy in measuring current disease prevalence trends or geographic differences in disease prevalence.

Figures 5.6 and 5.7 show the geographic distribution of reported case rates in fiscal years 1947 and 1965. Perhaps the most significant aspect of these two figures is the relative decrease of late and late latent syphilis rates in most of the southeastern states from 1947 to 1965, and the relative increase in reported disease prevalence in the Middle Atlantic States.

The Public Health Service believes that casefinding efforts in all states have succeeded for a number of years in finding more cases of syphilis than are occurring, thus reducing the prevalence or reservoir of disease. A great many of the detected and reported cases in past years were in the southeastern states. Due to the differential migration pattern of syphilitics and nonsyphilitics, and due to the definition of morbidity as being cases previously unreported in "this" state, an unknown number of cases previously detected and reported in the South are currently being detected and reported again in the northern states.

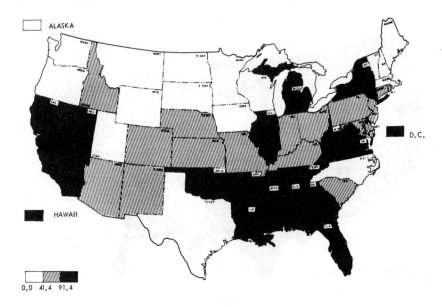

Fig. 5.6. Late and late latent syphilis case rates per 100,000 population: each state, fiscal year ending June 30, 1947.

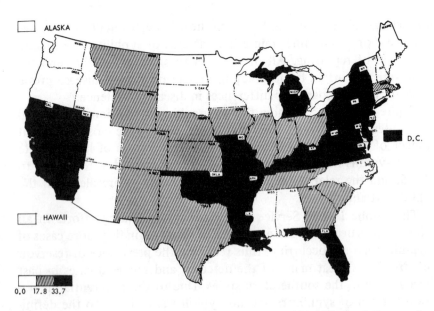

Fig. 5.7. Late and late latent syphilis case rates per 100,000 population: each state, fiscal year ending June 30, 1965.

The National Health Examination Survey, adjusting for differences among regions in the age, race, and sex composition of the population, found the highest rate of reactivity in the West, the lowest in the Northeast, and a middle range of reactivity rates in the South. This finding does not correlate with morbidity rates; however, the interpretation of rates of reactivity (for the most part persons who have or have had syphilis) and reported morbidity (cases previously unreported in a state) measure such diverse situations that neither is a reliable index of prevalence when defined as the number of cases which need treatment for syphilis.

Sex

The following tabulation gives the distribution of reported cases of syphilis in the United States in fiscal year 1966 by color, sex, and stage of disease:

Stage of syphilis	White		Nonwhite	
	Male	Female	Male	Female
Primary and secondary	3,567	1,169	10,163	7,574
Early latent	2,963	1,436	6,766	5,809
Late and late latent	16,772	13,133	18,814	17,430

In the infectious stage, the considerable excess of male over female cases is believed to be due more to missed diagnoses in the females because of often hidden primary symptoms than to an actual excess incidence among males. In the latent and late stages some of the excess of male cases disappears. The National Health Examination Survey, using a serologic test as an index of prevalence, found that 2.3 percent of their sample of white males were reactive to the KRP test for syphilis compared to 2.1 percent among white females and 22.9 percent reactive among Negro men compared to 16.3 percent among Negro women.[9] For all races 4.4 percent of men and 3.6 percent of women were reactive to the test for syphilis. Thus, the available data indicate a higher incidence and prevalence of syphilis among men than among women.

Race

The Public Health Service collects morbidity for the two color groups—white and nonwhite. The following United States morbidity data for fiscal year 1966 indicate that the syphilis rate (per 100,000 population) is several times higher among nonwhites than among whites:

Stage of syphilis	White		Nonwhite	
	Cases	Rate	Cases	Rate
Primary and secondary	4,736	2.8	17,737	76.1
Early latent	4,399	2.6	12,575	53.9
Total all stages	41,269	24.2	68,859	295.3

Caution should be exercised in the interpretation of color differences from morbidity statistics due to a probable color reporting bias. It is thought that relatively more nonwhite than white people avail themselves of health department clinics for medical services. Since public clinics report all of their cases of venereal disease, and since underreporting of disease occurs with private physicians, there is likely to be a reporting differential for white and nonwhite persons infected with syphilis. The amount of this reporting bias is not known.

The National Health Examination Survey reported the rate of reactivity to the KRP test for syphilis among white adults to be 2.2 percent and among Negroes to be 19.3 percent.[10] This would indicate syphilis to be about nine times as prevalent among Negroes as among whites compared to a reported morbidity rate for nonwhites which is 11 times as high as the white rate for all stages of syphilis.

Age

Syphilis is acquired almost exclusively during the young and middle adult period of life. As measured by reported cases of syphilis in the primary and secondary stage, only 1.1 percent of cases occurring in the United States in 1966 were among persons less than fifteen years of age, and only 3.3 percent of cases occurred among persons over fifty (Table 5.3). The 20-24 year age group, accounting for a little over one-fourth of all infectious cases, acquires syphilis more often than any other five-year age group, followed in order by the 25-29 and 15-19 year age groups. The 15-19 year age group accounted for approximately one out of every six acquired cases in 1966.

Table 5.3 Reported cases of primary and secondary syphilis by age, color, and sex: United States, 1966

Age group	Total Both Sexes Number	Percent	Total Male Number	Percent	Total Female Number	Percent	White Male Number	Percent	White Female Number	Percent	Nonwhite Male Number	Percent	Nonwhite Female Number	Percent
Total	21,414	100.0	12,997	100.0	8,417	100.0	3,244	100.0	1,170	100.0	9,753	100.0	7,247	100.0
0-14	242	1.1	69	.5	173	2.1	5	.2	7	.6	64	.7	166	2.3
15-19	3,846	18.0	1,731	13.3	2,115	25.1	239	7.4	227	19.4	1,492	15.3	1,888	26.1
20-24	6,033	28.2	3,509	27.0	2,524	30.0	749	23.1	325	27.8	2,760	28.3	2,199	30.3
25-29	4,339	20.3	2,835	21.8	1,504	17.9	656	20.2	217	18.5	2,179	22.3	1,287	17.8
30-39	4,485	20.9	3,047	23.4	1,438	17.1	913	28.1	243	20.8	2,134	21.9	1,195	16.5
40-49	1,752	8.2	1,258	9.7	494	5.9	448	13.8	111	9.5	810	8.3	383	5.3
50 and over	717	3.3	548	4.2	169	2.0	234	7.2	40	3.4	314	3.2	129	1.8

The results of the data presented in Table 5.3 indicate that non-whites acquire syphilis at a somewhat earlier age than whites, and females of both races at a somewhat earlier age than males.

Table A.I.20 shows cases and age specific rates of primary and secondary syphilis by color and sex for the years 1957, 1962, and 1965. Between 1957 and 1962 when infectious syphilis was increasing at a rate of as much as 50 percent per year in the United States, all age groups showed sharp increases in the incidence of syphilis. Although the reported incidence of syphilis for all ages increased between 1962 and 1965, there was a small and almost continuous decrease in the case rate for white persons under age thirty and nonwhites under age twenty-five. Much of the increases in infectious syphilis rates since 1962 are attributed to increases in the middle age and older part of the population.

Urban-Rural Distribution

Data presented in Table 5.4 compare fiscal year 1965 rates per 100,000 population for sixty-one cities of the United States with more than 200,000 population with the rates for the United States excluding these sixty-one cities.

Reported morbidity rates indicate that cities of more than 200,000 population have a venereal disease attack rate three to five times higher than smaller cities and rural areas.

The degree to which the disproportionate distribution of color groups among the major cities and other areas accounts for the difference in reported case rates is not known and investigation of this factor is beyond the scope of this monograph.

The Health Examination Survey of 1960-1962 using age, race, and sex adjusted rates of reactive serologic tests as a measurement of syphilis prevalence did not discern any urban-rural differences in prevalence.

Reported cases of syphilis and rates per 100,000 population for cities of more than 200,000 population for selected fiscal years are presented in Tables A.I.10-14. These data indicate that although there are large differences among cities in reported case rates, the trends of cases and rates in cities have been remarkably consistent with national trends.

Table 5.4 Number of cases and case rates per 100,000 population for syphilis and gonorrhea in total United States, 61 cities with more than 200,000 population, and rest of country, fiscal year 1965

Disease	United States Total	Major cities	U. S. excluding major cities
Syphilis			
All stages			
Cases	113,018	61,993	51,025
Rates	59.7	126.5	36.4
Primary and secondary			
Cases	23,250	11,417	11,833
Rates	12.3	23.3	8.4
Gonorrhea			
Cases	310,155	195,859	114,293
Rates	163.8	399.7	81.4

6 / Gonorrhea

Definition

Gonorrhea, a specific inflammation involving the mucous membrane of the genitourinary tract, is the predominant infection caused by the gonococcus *(Neisseria gonorrhoeae)*. Gonorrhea is the most prevalent of the venereal diseases and the most common bacterial infection of adults. The gonococcus may also cause extragenitourinary disease by spread from the primary focus. While the percentage of such complications is small, they are important because of the serious sequelae that frequently result.

Background

There is much evidence to suggest that gonorrhea is a disease of great antiquity. While not defined in modern terminology, ancient Egyptian, Hebrew, Chinese, and Greek references are highly suggestive of the presence of gonorrhea in those times. Leviticus 15 chronicles the management, including therapy and public health measures, to be invoked when confronted by a disease of venereal origin characterized by a discharge.

The term *gonorrhea* was coined by Galen in 130 A.D. and is translated literally as "a flow of seed." Accounts by Guillaume de Salicet and John of Arderne in the thirteenth and fourteenth centuries leave little doubt that the infection was not only prevalent and recognized as venereal in origin, but was also regarded as a separate and distinct disease entity.

The confusion between syphilis and gonorrhea appears to have developed almost immediately upon recognition of the former in the last years of the fifteenth century as epidemic syphilis swept Western Europe. A usually accurate observer, Paracelsus, taught in 1530 that gonorrhea was an initial symptom of syphilis. In that particularly unabashed and licentious era, multiple venereal infections were undoubtedly very common. Indeed, they are not rare today in this country and are not unusual in other countries where higher syphilis rates exist. However, not all physicians of that age were convinced about the inosculate nature of these diseases, and debate continued unabated until the tragic self-experimentation of John Hunter in

1767. Hunter obtained pus from a patient with gonorrhea and inoculated himself. Unfortunately, the inoculum was contaminated with the causative organism of syphilis and the development of both diseases followed in typical fashion. Despite mercurial therapy for cutaneous syphilids, Hunter developed classic syphilitic heart disease, which ultimately caused his death in 1793.

Hunter's reputation was such that, despite the experiments of Hill and Bell in the 1790's clearly differentiating the two diseases, most medical opinion held them to be the same for another half century. The credit for finally changing medical thought and delineating the two infections belongs to Philippe Ricord, who extensively studied the problem in the middle of the last century.

In 1879 Albert Neisser identified the causative organism in the purulent secretions of acute cases of urethritis and cervicitis and from the conjunctivae in cases of ophthalmia neonatorum. He referred to the organism as the "gonococcus." The organism was first cultivated by Leistikow in 1882. Bumm in 1885 was able to maintain the organism in pure culture and by inoculating volunteers fulfilled Koch's postulates. Two years after Neisser's discovery, Crede proved that gonococcal ophthalmia neonatorum could be prevented by the use of silver nitrate drops in the eyes of the newborn.

For centuries gonorrhea was treated with urethral irrigations and instillations. In the last century sandalwood oil was the standard therapeutic agent until potassium permanganate solution was introduced by Janet in 1892. Treatment with gonococcal vaccines, antitoxins, and filtrates were tried along with typhoid-paratyphoid vaccine, malaria, and other forms of fever therapy, all having advocates early in this century. In the latter part of the 1930's the effectiveness of the various sulfonamide preparations was demonstrated, and they readily gained ascendency over all other medications and local forms of therapy, which may have actually contributed to the complications of the disease. However, it had become obvious by the middle years of World War II that sulfonamides were no longer effective in many cases of gonorrhea. Penicillin appeared at this time and produced almost miraculous results which readily established it as the therapeutic agent of choice for all gonococcal infections. The lessons concerning the development of sulfonamide resistance were quickly forgotten as the penicillin success story established itself throughout the world.

Epidemiology

Gonorrhea in the United States remains a major public health problem. In the year ending June 30, 1941, state health departments reported a total of 193,468 cases of gonorrhea to the Public Health Service. The numbers of cases reported annually increased thereafter, reaching a peak of 400,639 cases in fiscal year 1947. Cases declined each year after 1947, reaching a low point of 216,448 in 1957, after which regular annual increases were reported again. In fiscal year 1965 state departments of health reported 310,155 cases of gonorrhea to the Public Health Service. While reporting remains poor, over 334,000 cases were reported in 1966,[1] and it is reliably estimated that at a minimum Americans are contracting gonorrhea at a rate exceeding 85,000 cases a month, or more than a million a year (Figure 6.1). In 1962 the results of a nationwide survey indicated that less than 10 percent of the gonorrhea cases treated by private physicians were reported to health officials.[2]

There is a great deal of variance in the reported incidence of gonorrhea among the states, the areas of high and low incidence correlating well with the geographic distribution of syphilis incidence. Table A.I.9 shows the state distribution of cases and rates for fiscal years 1941-1966.

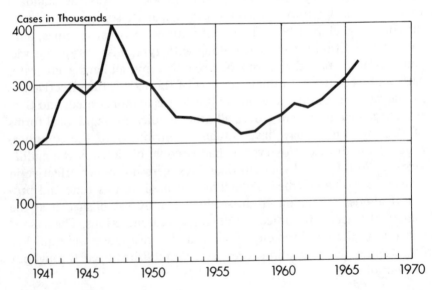

Fig. 6.1. Reported gonorrhea cases: United States, fiscal years ending June 30, 1941 to 1966.

No racial or individual immunity has been demonstrated, and the disease has a universal distribution. The World Health Organization officially estimates that sixty-five million new cases occur on a global basis each year.[3]

Transmission of the gonococcus is almost wholly by sexual intercourse and survival of the organism depends entirely on sexual promiscuity. Man is the only reservoir and known host. Throughout recorded medical history the incidence of gonorrhea, as well as other venereal diseases, traditionally rises during periods of war, migration, economic depression, or when other forms of social unrest become prevalent. As would be expected, the age of incidence of gonorrhea mirrors the age of greatest sexual activity. One half of reported cases occur in persons twenty-five years of age or younger.

Sex specific rates for gonorrhea (Table A.I.3.) indicate the disease to have three times as great an incidence among males as among females. This apparent difference between males and females is probably considerably exaggerated due to ease of diagnosis of the disease in the male, the difficulty of making a positive diagnosis in the female, and frequent lack of symptoms which would motivate females to seek diagnosis.

Color differences in incidence are just as great for gonorrhea as for syphilis. In fiscal year 1965 the reported gonorrhea rate in the United States was 999.2 per 100,000 nonwhite population compared to a rate of 51.6 per 100,000 white population (Table A.I.3.). Racial differences as indicated from morbidity data should be interpreted cautiously since there may be a reporting bias caused by greater utilization of health department diagnostic facilities by nonwhites than by whites. Since health department clinics report all diagnosed cases, a greater proportion of nonwhite cases would be reported.

The distribution of gonorrhea cases by age is almost identical to the distribution of early syphilis cases. The age distribution of cases and age specific rates by color and sex for the United States, years 1952, 1957 and 1965, are given in Table A.I.21.

Whether the increasing incidence of gonorrhea in younger persons, particularly teenagers, is related to increasing promiscuity within this group is debatable. However, it should be emphasized that the increase is not confined to the younger group, but affects all ages. Certainly public attitudes concerning gonorrhea which stem from apathy and ignorance remain casual and cavalier, hindering control. Treatment is not infrequently administered by unqualified persons or friends, eliminating any chance at identifying infected sexual contacts.

Several factors inherent in the natural history of gonorrhea further contribute to its continued ability to flourish. A very short incubation period, in contrast to that of syphilis, allows an extremely rapid spread. Unfortunately, an attack of gonorrhea produces little, if any, immunity to subsequent infections and repeat attacks are extremely common.

Another obstacle is the basically asymptomatic nature of the disease in females. It is seldom realized that upwards of 90 percent of females with gonorrhea are completely without symptoms and unaware that they are infected. This carrier state provides a large reservoir which remains undetected by current diagnostic and public health methods. A similar asymptomatic state probably also occurs in a small percentage of males.[4] In addition it can no longer be denied that the sensitivity of *N. gonorrhoeae* to penicillin is decreasing at a significant rate, and larger dosages of penicillin are now necessary for cure.[5] This aspect of the problem is further considered in the section on therapy.

Reports of nonvenereal transmission resulting in vulvovaginitis in prepubescent girls were once fairly commonplace. The diagnosis of gonorrhea in young girls should never be made on the basis of smear alone, but complete bacteriologic studies must be insisted upon. Most cases of vulvovaginitis are not gonococcal in origin or, if they are proved to be, persistent questioning and investigation will usually reveal that sexual contact or child molestation has occurred.

Bacteriology

In typical smears of urethral exudate, gonococci appear as intracellular gram-negative diplococci with flattened adjacent sides resembling a pair of coffee beans. Frequently single cocci, measuring 0.6 to 1.0 micron in diameter, are present extracellularly, particularly in very early or chronic infections. In smears, the distribution of organisms is very irregular, with most polymorphonuclear leukocytes containing no organisms while the much rarer actively phagocytic cells usually contain dozens of cocci. In smears taken from pure culture the organism may appear as a single coccus, typical diplococci, tetrads, or even larger clusters. The gonococcus is nonmotile, nonspore forming, and lacks a true capsule. Numerous other microorganisms found in the urogenital tract of man, particularly staphylococci, streptococci, certain diplobacilli, members of the tribe Mimeae and other Neisseria species may make the microscopic diagnosis difficult. This is especially true in the female where 3-10 percent harbor other Neisseria, most commonly *N. sicca* or *N. subflava.*[6]

While gonococci stain readily with most dyes, preparations made with polychrome stains or methylene blue may lead to confusion and should not be used in diagnosis. After more tham eighty years the Gram stain remains the staining method of choice. Smears from the conjunctivae or from secretions of the female urogenital tract are not fully reliable due to the frequent presence of other gram-negative cocci. Dead staphylococci frequently are observed to be gram-negative and other varieties of rapidly dividing organisms may have diplococcal morphology and atypical staining, leading to additional confusion. For these reasons and because of the time involved in searching gram stained smears with few or no gonococci present, this method of diagnosis should be abandoned in favor of the more definitive culture and fluorescent antibody techniques except in cases of typical male urethritis. Smears obtained from patients who have received treatment with penicillin or other antibiotics may show organisms with profoundly altered appearance. The cocci progressively enlarge and become less stainable until they are no longer recognizable or detectable.

The gonococcus is a fastidious organism, and primary isolation requires the addition of undefined complex organic substances such as ascitic fluid, plasma, hemoglobin, or whole blood. Some peptones contain concentrations of amino acids which are toxic to gonococcal growth. Heating the media after the addition of whole blood results in chocolate agar which is much less toxic. Toxic fatty acid substances encountered in some lots of agar may be neutralized by the addition of charcoal or starch to the media.

Despite the wide availability of commercial media and supplements, cultural identification remained for many years an arduous, painstaking procedure requiring considerable bacteriologic sophistication. The identification of *N. gonorrhoeae* has in recent years been greatly simplified by the introduction of two new basic techniques.

In 1959 the first of these new tools was developed by applying fluorescent antibody (FA) procedures to the problem of gonococcal identification. Stemming from this application the following diagnostic tests were developed: immediate direct FA, delayed direct FA,[7] and rapid immunofluorescent staining.[8] In acute male gonorrhea any of these FA methods are equal to culture or Gram stain in sensitivity. However, at least in diagnostic situations, the FA procedures are virtually specific for *N. gonorrhoeae* and are thus preferable to Gram staining methods.

In female patients who are known contacts of males with gonorrhea the number of organisms is frequently small and the immediate direct FA procedure will be positive in only 30 percent of cases. By culturing negative specimens for 16 hours and then performing the direct FA procedure, the positivity rate is increased to approximately 50-60 percent. The additional culture increases the number of organisms and thereby the sensitivity. A rapid immunofluorescent staining procedure requiring only one minute to perform has recently been developed but is in need of further evaluation. It has also been suggested that the addition of counterstains such as flazo-orange[9] or Evan's blue dye[10] to the staining procedure will help eliminate the problem of background fluorescence and improve the performance of the FA procedures.

Interest in the FA diagnostic techniques has diminished since the introduction by Thayer and Martin of two antibiotic-containing media selective for the pathogenic *Neisseria*. The first Thayer-Martin medium (T-M) described contained ristocetin and polymyxin B.[11] More recently a second medium (VCN) containing sodium colistimethate, vancomycin, and nystatin has been described.[12] The results obtained with these media when specimens are taken from heavily contaminated sites such as the vagina or rectum far surpass the best performance of conventional media. The new VCN media is actually superior to the original antibiotic formulation, because it is slightly less inhibitory for the gonococcus than the older ristocetin-polymyxin supplement while inhibiting a wider range of saprophytic organisms.

When appropriate specimens are plated on antibiotic media and the resulting colonies have typical morphology, a positive oxidase reaction with 1 percent dimethyl-p-phenylenediamine hydrochloride, and characteristic Gram stain reaction, the presumptive diagnosis of *N. gonorrhoeae* is virtually equivalent to a definitive diagnosis which requires secondary sugar fermentation reactions. Confirmatory fermentation reactions with glucose should naturally be performed in cases involving minors, sexual assault, divorce, or other possible medicolegal situations.

The gonococcus is quickly destroyed by desiccation and clinical specimens must be carefully handled to maximize recovery chances. Should immediate plating be impossible, the swab or loop may be rinsed into a small volume of broth (2ml) and stored at 4° for a few hours prior to subsequent culture. Although the gonococcus is an aerobic organism, many strains require an atmosphere of 2 percent to 10 percent CO_2 to initiate growth. The ordinary candle extinction jar conveniently provides this atmosphere. The optimum temperature for incubation is between 35°C and 36°C.

Attempts to infect experimental animals, including anthropoid apes, with the gonococcus have been notoriously unsuccessful despite the efforts of many competent investigators. The gonococcus does possess an endotoxin, similar in nature to that of the meningococcus, which will kill laboratory animals when injected in sufficient amounts, but death is obviously not due to infection. Two strains, now both lost, have been reported which produced fatal infections when injected intraperitoneally with mucin into the mouse.[13] Local infections involving the anterior chamber of the rabbit eye have also been reported.[14]

Symptoms and Signs

Because the gonococcus is unable to penetrate normal skin, initial infection develops only on those surfaces lined with mucous membrane tissue. Primary infection usually involves the male urethra, the cervix, the ducts of Bartholin's glands, the paraurethral ducts of either sex or the rectal mucosa. The eye is also an occasional primary site. On rare occasions the immature and hence susceptible lining of the vagina in prepubescent females may be the site of primary infection.

In males the usual incubation period of natural infection is two to five days. The incubation period may be much longer and several weeks may elapse before symptoms are noted. Typically, patients have a sudden onset of frequent, painful urination accompanied by a profuse mucopurulent urethral discharge. After a variable period infection spreads to the posterior urethra, prostate, seminal vesicles, and epididymis. Acute prostatitis is manifested by pelvic pain, fever, and occasionally urinary retention. Epididymitis is characterized by severe pain, tenderness, and swelling. Careful palpation will reveal that the testicle is not actually involved. Following adequate treatment, symptomatic improvement is prompt, urethritis usually subsiding within twenty-four hours. Prostatitis and epididymitis respond more slowly, and the possibility of sterility resulting from the latter complication should not be forgotten.

Most females with gonorrhea are asymptomatic, and the diagnosis is based on bacteriologic evidence or the history of contact with an infected male. A small minority of women may complain of vaginal discharge or urinary frequency and pain. Profuse leukorrhea is rarely gonococcal in origin. Bartholinitis is not common and most Bartholin abscesses are due to organisms other than the gonococcus. When involved, the ducts of Bartholin's glands may be reddened, and the glands themselves are painful and enlarged.

Pelvic inflammatory disease occurs when spread from the cervical glands to the fallopian tubes takes place. This diagnosis is primarily one of exclusion. Fever, nausea, vomiting, and lower abdominal pain often appear suddenly, simulating appendicitis or other acute surgical conditions. Peritoneal signs may appear. A history of sexual exposure and the demonstration of gonococci on stained smears of cervical secretions are helpful if positive. However, the diagnosis of definite gonococcal etiology cannot be made on this basis unless supported by more definite bacteriological findings. Surgical consultation should be sought in cases where the diagnosis remains obscure, and exploratory laporotomy may be necessary on occasion to establish the diagnosis. Frequently, salpingitis recurs in repeated episodes marked by pain and fever. Usually, it cannot be established whether this is due to reinfection or reactivation of incompletely sterilized foci of infection.

Gonococcal septicemia may result in several important clinical syndromes. While no longer common, these metastatic infections are increasing in incidence accompanying the general increase in gonorrhea. Prompt recognition is important, because early therapy may prevent residual morbidity. It should be remembered that a primary urogenital focus of infection may not be obvious since these patients are often asymptomatic. Carefully conducted bacteriologic studies are frequently necessary to locate the initial site of infection.

The most common extragenital complication is arthritis, which may occur at any time following the initial infection. This condition was observed in 3-5 percent of patients with gonorrhea in the preantibiotic era, but now is much reduced in incidence. Females are more commonly affected than males, most modern series reporting at least a 2:1 ratio. The onset of symptoms frequently occurs during or immediately following the menses. Over 25 percent of cases occur during pregnancy or in the immediate post partum period. The onset usually is sudden with chills, high fever, and migratory polyarthralgia. More rarely the condition may be present in a subacute fashion with stiffness, swelling, tenderness, and pain in one or more joints. The majority of patients have two or more joints involved. The joints most commonly affected are the knees, ankles, hips, and wrists, but any joint may be involved. Tenosynovitis (inflammation of a tendon sheath) is a common accompaniment of gonococcal arthritis and is seen in over three-quarters of all cases. The presence of tenosynovitis involving the tendons of the wrists, hands, or ankles provides a valuable diagnostic sign, because it is far more common in this condition than in other forms of arthritis. Skin lesions are not uncommon and may be either hemorrhagic or vesiculopustular in type. The skin of the extremities, particularly the palms and soles, are the sites of predilection.[15] These lesions are usually tender and sparse; they involute in four to five days. Successful culture of gonococci from skin lesions has been reported but is a rare event.

The diagnosis of gonococcal arthritis may be difficult since gonococci are recovered from an aspirate of joint fluid in only about 25 percent of cases. The presumptive diagnosis is based on the recovery of the organism from a urogenital site, the clinical findings, and the response to antibiotic therapy. The differential diagnosis includes rheumatoid arthritis, other forms of pyogenic arthritis, serum sickness, rheumatic fever, Reiter's disease, and gout.

Meningitis is a severe and rare complication of gonococcemia. The symptomatology is similar to other forms of pyogenic meningitis and the diagnosis depends entirely upon the laboratory identification of the organism. The organisms recovered from about 2 percent of diagnosed meningococcal meningitis cases have actually been shown to be *N. gonorrhoeae* when appropriate sugar fermentation tests are applied.

Gonococcal endocarditis is another rare complication of gonorrhea. The course is fulminating and frequently fatal. The valves of the left side of the heart are most frequently involved. Repeated blood cultures are usually necessary to establish the diagnosis since the bacteremia is transient and ordinary media may not support the growth of this fastidious organism.

Gonococcal conjunctivitis in adults may result from gonococcemia or more frequently from direct inoculation via fingers contaminated with infectious genital secretions. An extremely purulent and destructive conjunctivitis is produced. Both topical and parentereal antibiotics started immediately upon diagnosis are essential if corneal perforation and residual blindness are to be prevented.

Other very rare features of metastatic gonorrhea include uveitis, myocarditis, pericarditis, cystitis, glomerulonephritis, perihepatitis, liver abscesses, myositis, osteomyelitis, and pneumonia.

Diagnosis

In the male the presence of gram-negative intracellular diplococci in urethral pus combined with typical clinical symptoms is virtually diagnostic. Organisms of the *Mima-Herellea* group have been mistaken for gonococci on microscopic examination of Gram stained smears. However, these organisms are encountered in urethritis patients so infrequently in this country that confusion on this basis rarely results. These organisms may be easily differentiated by their growth on unenriched media and inhibition by selective media. If no discharge is present, a smear or preferably a culture may be made from the sediment obtained by centrifuging the first 10 ml. of voided urine or from prostate secretions following prostatic massage. The first voided morning urine specimen is preferred and delays in handling must be avoided since urine is toxic for gonococci. In cases where the organisms are not typical or absent on Gram stain, nongonococcal urethritis must be ruled out by cultural procedures.

To maximize the possibility of diagnosis, female patients should ideally have cervical, vaginal, urethral, and rectal specimens taken for culture. However, for practical purposes cervical and rectal cultures suffice. Vaginal cultures almost entirely reflect gonococci shed from the cervix and are frequently heavily contaminated with other microorganisms. Routine culture of the urethra is rarely productive since coexisting cervical infection is almost invariably associated and only rarely will the urethra alone be found positive. It is important to realize that in approximately 10 percent of infected females only the rectal site yields positive cultures.[16] If only a single site is selected for culture the cervix should be chosen since about 85 percent of infected patients will harbor organisms at this site. The cervical mucous plug should be carefully removed and the actual specimens taken from the walls of the endocervical canal following repeated gentle massage of the cervix between the blades of a bivalve vaginal speculum. The speculum should be lubricated with warm water only because many lubricants contain bactericidal substances. For best results the exudates should be inoculated directly since the number of organisms is frequently small. Rectal specimens are preferably taken from the rectal crypts following direct visualization with a proctoscope. It is generally preferable to collect all specimens with a small platinum loop instead of cotton swabs. This is especially helpful in female patients where the amount of exudate is often limited. It is worth emphasizing that Gram stained smears are unreliable in the diagnosis of gonorrhea in the female and should not be used for this purpose.

All materials collected from the female urogenital tracts are preferably cultured on selective media due to the likelihood of contamination. Isolation of gonococci from rectal sites is particularly facilitated by the use of selective media. Studies have shown that even when specimens are obtained from relatively uncontaminated areas such as the male urethra or endocervix, higher isolation rates are obtained with selective media.[17, 18] Fluorescent antibody procedures, especially the delayed technique, are also quite useful for diagnosis. These techniques require quite skilled laboratory personnel for successful application and in general the results, while approaching those of selective culture, are inferior.

Blood, joint aspirates, or other body fluids should be cultured in flasks containing glucose-ascitic fluid broth and then subcultured on suitably enriched chocolate agar. Penicillinase should be added to the broth to a final concentration of 1.0 unit per ml. if the patient has been receiving this antibiotic.

Whenever possible, laboratory personnel should be alerted that the gonococcus is suspected so that optimum techniques and conditions for isolation will be utilized.

Except on an experimental basis serologic tests for gonorrhea are no longer available in the United States. The complement-fixation reaction utilizing gonococcal antigen was widely utilized in the years preceding World War II, but interest in this procedure has diminished in the intervening years. The demise of the procedure resulted from an apparent lack of specificity and undersensitivity.

Since the vast asymptomatic female reservoir is unaffected by present control measures, it is agreed that a serologic test readily applicable to large scale detection of the disease would represent real progress in gonorrhea control. Therefore, renewed interest in the complement-fixation technique and the application of other immunological testing procedures to the gonorrhea problem has developed in the past several years. Several promising techniques have been reported, but to date none has received wide acceptance.[19, 20, 21]

Therapy

Recent years have seen an escalation in the dosages of penicillin required to cure gonorrhea. This relative "resistance" by the gonococcus to penicillin was little more than a laboratory curiosity less than a decade ago. At that time "resistant" strains which arbitrarily require 0.1 unit of penicillin per ml. for *in vitro* inhibition were extremely rare in clinical practice. Such strains are commonplace today. Present evidence indicates that considerable geographic variation exists regarding the distribution of these strains. Certain areas, both abroad and within the United States, have not as yet experienced the impact of this problem. In this country eastern cities report fewer infections with "resistant" gonococci than midwestern or western cities. From the latter, strains requiring 0.5 unit per ml. of penicillin for *in vitro* inhibition are now common. Due to the increasing mobility of the population there is no doubt that these more "resistant" strains will become more widely disseminated.

Despite this problem penicillin remains the drug of choice in gonorrhea. When infection is caused by a gonococcus with lessened susceptibility to penicillin, high blood levels, usually three to ten times the *in vitro* minimum inhibitory concentration, are required for cure. To achieve necessary blood levels, short-acting penicillin preparations are required. Hence, along with increasing dosages there has been an accompanying shift to short-acting penicillins. In the past gonorrhea was widely and successfully treated with long-acting penicillins but many authorities feel this practice has been responsible for the decline in gonococcal sensitivity. Reinfection in patients maintaining subinhibitory penicillin levels would seemingly provide ideal conditions for the development of resistance. Benzathine penicillin or other long acting preparations should not be used in the hope of preventing reinfection or as an antibiotic quarantine since reinfection is actually only delayed and not prevented. Such penicillin preparations, while ideal in syphilis, have no place in the treatment of gonorrhea.

Uncomplicated gonococcal urethritis in the male is adequately treated with 2,400,000 units of aqueous procaine penicillin G (APPG) in a single intramuscular injection. Females require higher doses if a satisfactory cure rate is to be obtained, and 4,800,000 units of APPG or a mixture of 2,400,000 units of APPG and 2,400,000 units of aqueous procaine penicillin G in oil with aluminum monostearate are currently recommended.[22] Usually this amount of penicillin is divided and given at two injection sites during a single visit. Patients of either sex failing on this therapy should be retreated with double the original dose given over a period of one or two days. Gonococcal proctitis is treated in the same manner as urethritis or cervicitis and usually does not require additional therapy.

Urethritis patients frequently will complain of a slight watery or mucoid discharge following therapy. This discharge is felt by many to represent a nongonococcal urethritis contracted simultaneously with the gonorrhea. More likely explanations are that it is due to subsiding urethral inflammation or is caused by a temporary overgrowth of antibiotic resistant organisms residing within the urethra. Various yeasts or staphylococcus albus are frequently cultured from such discharges. After ruling out relapse or reinfection by culture, further therapy is not indicated as it may only prolong the discharge which usually spontaneously subsides within a week or ten days. Patients should be cautioned against undue self-examination by urethral stripping since this practice may result in a mechanical urethritis.

Gonococcal epididymitis, seminal vesiculitis, and prostatitis are usually satisfactorily treated with 2,400,000 units of APPG daily for five to seven days. Patients with acute gonococcal salpingitis require bed rest and high dosages of parenteral penicillin. Crystalline penicillin G given by intravenous infusion or intramuscular APPG injections (equally divided and spaced) totaling 5,000,000 to 10,000,000 units per day for seven to fourteen days is recommended. Surgery is not indicated during the acute episode unless abscess formation occurs and requires drainage. The response to penicillin is usually prompt with pain and fever subsiding within twenty-four to forty-eight hours. In chronic cases where periodic episodes of salpingitis recur, eventual surgical excision of the involved organs may be necessary. Such surgery should be limited to carefully selected patients in whom recurrences are of sufficient frequency and severity to seriously interfere with the patient's comfort or livelihood.

Unfortunately, in most cases scar formation has already resulted in closure of infected tubes and the patient is sterile.

Gonococcal vulvovaginitis in children is treated in the same fashion as adult urethritis but with reduced dosage depending upon the patient's age and weight.

Gonococcal arthritis usually responds dramatically to bed rest and penicillin. Crystalline penicillin given by the intravenous route totaling 8,000,000 to 12,000,000 units per day for fourteen days is recommended. If adequate treatment is begun early in the course of the disease, no residual joint damage should result. Thick pus, when present, should be aspirated, but intracavitary penicillin is not indicated, because diffusion readily occurs into joints.

Gonococcal meningitis or endocarditis are life-threatening infections and large doses of parenteral penicillin G over prolonged periods are essential. From 10,000,000 to 20,000,000 units daily are suggested. The treatment of meningitis usually requires ten to fourteen days and endocarditis from four to six weeks.

Ophthalmia neonatorum and gonococcal conjunctivitis in the adult require both parenteral and topical penicillin. In infants, 300,000 to 600,000 units of APPG administered parenterally daily are recommended. In adults the parenteral dose is that for urethritis. Both adults and children should have local instillations of penicillin G in physiological saline (10,000 units per ml.) repeated every two to four hours until the infection clears.

Penicillin-sensitive patients with uncomplicated gonorrhea may be treated with a tetracycline or erythromycin, 0.5 gm orally every four hours until 3.0 gm have been given. Most male patients will also respond well to a single oral dose of 1.5 gm of tetracycline. Patients with urogenital or metastatic complications should be given tetracycline or erythromycin, 0.5 gm orally every six hours for seven to fourteen days.

Tests of cure are ordinarily not necessary in males since the cessation of symptoms is usually tantamount to cure. However, such tests are essential in the proper management of gonorrhea in the female. Specimens should be collected for culture on selective media from all sites originally found infected. When short acting penicillins have been used in therapy, cultures may be made one week following treatment and if possible for two more weekly intervals. There is no definite evidence that gonococci in the rectum, despite the coexistence of penicillinase-producing organisms, are harder to eradicate than gonococci at other sites.

It should not be forgotten that gonorrhea patients may also have contracted syphilis and can be incubating that infection while under treatment for gonorrhea. The effects of current gonorrhea therapy recommendations upon incubating syphilis are unknown but may not be curative. If not aborted, the incubation period may be prolonged beyond normal limits. Therefore, the proper management of gonorrhea dictates a base line serologic test for syphilis when gonorrhea is diagnosed and subsequent monthly serologic tests for a minimum period of four months.

7 / Mortality Caused by Syphilis and Its Sequelae and Other Late Manifestations of Untreated Venereal Disease

Classification of Cause of Death

Statistics on causes of death are derived from the medical certification of causes of death prepared by the attending physician or by a coroner in cases of death by violence or where a medical practitioner was not in attendance. The medical information so reported on the death certificate is classified according to the *International Statistical Classification of Diseases, Injuries, and Causes of Death* (ISC). This classification scheme provides a uniform basis for the classification of causes of death.

During the period for which mortality statistics are shown in this report, the causes of death were classified according to seven different revisions of the ISC. To keep abreast of medical knowledge, it has been the practice to revise the ISC every ten years since 1900. Each decennial revision has produced some break in the comparability of cause of death statistics. For the most part, the degree of discontinuity in the trend has not been considered a great problem.

The effects of changes in the classification of death on the cause of death statistics have been described by Van Buren up to the 1938 Revision.[1] Dunn and Shackley compared the cause of death assignments by the 1929 and 1938 Revisions of the ISC.[2] Comparable category numbers between the Fifth and Sixth Revisions of the ISC have been published by the Vital Statistics Division, National Center for Health Statistics.[3]

One problem in comparing death rates by cause of death over a time period spanning sixty-three years is the selection of a list of causes for which comparable data are available. In some instances, a comparable group of causes may be established by regrouping rubrics tabulated according to an earlier revision to correspond with changes made in the grouping of terms by the subsequent revision. However, when a new term was not previously identified in the ISC, or a term was not tabulated separately in one revision but was reassigned in the next revision, no adjustment in data is possible.

Essentially comparable causes of death used in each revision and the category numbers used to code syphilis and its sequelae through seven revisions of the ISC are shown in Table A.II.1.

Of course, comparability between revisions cannot be evaluated by comparing category numbers alone. It is necessary to consider the inclusion terms as shown under each title in the ISC for that revision.

Changes in diagnostic practice, in reporting practice, in completing the death certificate, and in the coding practice used to select the cause of death to be tabulated are also important.

There have been some changes in the assignment of various conditions to syphilis as a cause of death between each of the revisions of the ISC. The assignment of deaths caused by aneurysm of the aorta has presented a particular problem. For the First and Second Revisions, 1900-1920, deaths from aneurysm were not separately classified and could not be tabulated either as a whole or in part. For the Third and Fourth Revisions, 1921-1938, deaths from aneurysm of the aorta were tabulated with aneurysm (except of heart) and included with syphilis tabulations in this report. However, prior to 1939 aneurysm had little weight in the *Manual of Joint Causes of Death* and was frequently tabulated under associated causes. In the Fifth Revision, 1939-1948, and for the years 1949-1954 of the Sixth Revision, deaths from aneurysm of the aorta were tabulated with deaths from syphilis, except when the aneurysm was specified as nonsyphilitic in origin. Some important changes were introduced in the 1955 *Instruction, Manual for Cause of Death Coding.*[4] For the remainder of the Sixth Revision, 1955-1957, and for the Seventh Revision, 1958-1963, deaths from aneurysm of the aorta were tabulated with deaths from syphilis only if specified as syphilitic in origin.

The Sixth Revision, first used in 1949, represented a more sweeping change than any of the previous revisions. The classification scheme was expanded considerably to provide specific categories for nonfatal diseases and for nature of injury. In the process of expansion, provision was made to permit comparability of certain categories with important titles of the Fifth Revision of the ISC. However, strict comparability for mortality between the two revisions is lost because of some regrouping of the titles necessary in the Sixth Revision to accommodate the causes of morbidity.

In addition to the changes in the classification list itself, selecting the cause of death for primary mortality tabulations was modified considerably in 1949. When only one cause of death is reported on the death certificate, the assignment of the cause of death is simple. However, in this century as medical diagnosis has become increasingly more sophisticated, multiple factors are frequently reported on the death certificate. The method used to determine the one cause to which the death will be assigned has an important effect upon the resulting statistics.

Before 1949, when more than one cause was reported, the selection of a cause of death for tabulation was made by reference to a fixed set of priority tables published in the *Manual of Joint Causes of Death*. The joint-cause rules were also revised periodically. The rules adopted with the Sixth Revision, used in 1949 and in subsequent years, specify that where the medical certification is properly completed, the underlying cause of death indicated by the physician shall be accepted for tabulation.

When comparing syphilis mortality statistics for the years prior to and subsequent to 1949, one must take into consideration the changes in the classification lists and the method used to select the underlying cause of death for primary mortality tabulations.

To measure the net effect of changes in the assignment of various conditions by cause, the International Conference for the Sixth Decennial Revision of the ISC recommended that the deaths reported in one year should be coded according to both the Fifth and Sixth Revisions. In the United States, deaths reported during 1950 were coded according to both the Fifth and the Sixth Revisions.[5]

The comparability ratio is a factor obtained by dividing the number of deaths assigned to a particular cause using one revision by the number of deaths assigned to that cause by another revision. For syphilis deaths, the comparability ratio between the Fifth and Sixth Revisions is 0.72. In other words, 28 percent fewer deaths were assigned to syphilis and its sequelae when the cause of death was classified according to the Sixth Revision as compared with the same data classified according to the Fifth Revision.

The comparability ratio gives an indication of the net change between revisions. Comparability ratios vary with age at death and with color and sex, and, therefore, comparability ratios for total deaths due to syphilis cannot be applied to data specific for age, color, and sex. In addition, comparability ratios vary by state. Hence, comparability ratios for the United States cannot be applied to data by state. The comparability ratios for syphilis and its sequelae, by age, color, and sex for the Fifth and Sixth Revisions, United States, are shown in Table A.II.2.

In the majority of cases, application of the rules for the Seventh Revision, adopted for use in 1958, results in the same code assignment as that of the Sixth Revision rules. An increase of 3.3 percent for syphilis and its sequelae (020-029) occurred in 1958 by reason of a change in interpretation of aneurysm of the aorta reported in a sequence involving arteriosclerosis of sites other than the aorta.[6] It should be noted, however, that the interpretation of such sequences reverted in 1959 to that used with the Sixth Revision. Hence, the comparability ratio of 1.03 for this cause is applicable only to the year 1958.[7]

Reported Mortality from Syphilis

The reported deaths from syphilis are influenced by the prevalence of syphilis, the treatment of infections, the primary cause of death due to other causes, the difficulty of diagnosing syphilis as a cause of death, and the willingness of physicians to report syphilis as a cause of death when they have made the diagnosis.

The method of selecting the underlying cause of death affects the reported syphilis mortality rate. Beginning in 1949 the physician's statement regarding the underlying cause of death was accepted for tabulation. This procedure alone reduced reported syphilis deaths 28 percent. The joint-cause preference used in the Fifth Revision gave a high priority to syphilis, while apparently in many cases the physician certifying the cause of death described syphilis as a contributing cause rather than as the underlying cause of death.

Syphilis as a cause of death may be difficult to diagnose. This is particularly true of cardiovascular syphilis in patients not seen by the physician before death. A study of 8,182 autopsies in Germany (1928-1936) showed that the clinical diagnosis of syphilis as the cause of death was increased 26 percent (tabes dorsalis increased 63 percent and syphilitic aneurysm increased 250 percent) when verified by postmortem examination.[8] However, this study was published in 1937, and there have been many changes in medicine since that time. In 1937, for instance, 36.7 percent of all deaths occurred in hospitals or institutions; by 1958 more than 60 percent of all deaths occurred in hospitals or institutions. It seems reasonable to expect that the increasing availability of medical facilities and technology would tend to increase the accuracy of medical diagnosis.

Syphilis has been shown to be an accompanying or accessory cause of death twice as frequently by autopsy as by clinical examination.[9] During 1958, autopsies (in the United States) were reported on 32.1 percent of the deaths due to syphilis compared to only 19.1 percent autopsies for all causes. For major diseases of the heart, only 11.9 percent were reported with autopsies.[10] Thus, a relatively high percentage of syphilis as a cause of death depends upon an autopsy. Yet, almost 90 percent of the deaths attributed to major diseases of the heart are based on clinical diagnoses. The extent to which this factor affects reported syphilis deaths is not known.

Multiple cause of death tabulations provide some information on the extent to which a given disease is listed as a secondary or contributory cause in fatal cases to another disease. Information on multiple (or associated) causes of death was compiled on a sample of death certificates reported during 1955.[11] A total of 2,911,034 conditions were reported for 1,527,691 deaths in 1955. Fifty-eight percent of the medical certificates contained information on more than one cause of death.

During 1955 syphilis was listed as an associated cause of death 2,405 times. Although there were some changes in coding procedure between 1940 and 1955, the 1955 data contrasts sharply with the data tabulated during 1940 when syphilis was coded as an associated cause of death only 788 times out of a total of 1,417,269 deaths.[12] In some cases, perhaps penicillin treatment introduced about 1945 made a difference in reported deaths from syphilis by removing syphilis as the primary cause of death, thus making it a contributory cause of death.

During 1955 when syphilis was listed as an associated cause of death, it was most often listed with diseases of the circulatory system (45 percent of the total times listed); neoplasms (nearly 12 percent of the total times listed); diseases of the nervous system and sense organs (10 percent of the total times listed); and with diseases of the respiratory system (about 10 percent of the total times listed).[13] (See Table A.II.3.)

During 1955 syphilis was noted on the death certificate 6,735 times. In 3,825 instances syphilis was coded as the underlying cause of death. Thus, syphilis was an important factor in causing death 1.76 more times than the number of times it was recorded as the primary cause. Syphilis was listed somewhat more often as a contributory cause of death among the white population (male, 1.93; female, 1.73) than among the nonwhite population (male, 1.56; female, 1.50). General paralysis of the insane was listed as an associated cause of death 2.4 more times than it was listed as the primary cause of death. (See Table A.II.4.) These data attest to the fact that syphilis is an important factor in causing a number of deaths above and beyond the number of times it is recorded as the underlying cause of death.

It is realized that the recorded mortality rate from syphilis may not be synonymous with the real mortality from syphilis. In studies it has been shown that the reported mortality rate from syphilis may range as low as 51 percent[14] and 79 percent[15] of the true mortality from syphilis. However, there is a lack of current national statistics on the accuracy of medical diagnoses.

The factors influencing reported syphilis mortality indicate that syphilis is probably underreported as the underlying cause of death and that it is an important contributory factor as a cause of death in many instances. However, the extent to which these factors actually influenced the reporting of syphilis as the underlying cause of death is unknown.

Statistical trends in mortality by cause are affected by many factors including the level of diagnostic acumen, the care with which the death records are completed, and the classification used to code causes of death for tabulation. With regard to these data the same classification was used for all records in any given year, and therefore should not introduce any statistical bias between two population groups from this source. However, this consistency does not apply invariably in considering mortality trends which involve more than one revision of the *International Statistical Classification of Diseases, Injuries, and Causes of Death* (ISC). There are no comprehensive measures of the level of diagnostic acumen and completeness of records over a period of decades. Presumably diagnosis and registration have improved, but the relative degree of improvement for the various population groups, especially the white and nonwhite groups, remains unknown. Despite the many factors that complicate the interpretation of these data, they furnish a useful record of the changing patterns of mortality.

The Expected Outcome of Untreated Syphilis

The actual importance of syphilis as a cause of death is unknown. Information is needed on questions such as: To what extent does syphilis as a cause of death masquerade as other diseases? To what extent is syphilis an indirect cause of death from other diseases? What is the ultimate outcome if syphilis is not treated?

The fate of approximately 2,000 syphilitic patients who had received no specific therapy during the twenty-year period 1891-1910 in Oslo, Norway, was studied by Boeck and Bruusgaard. As noted in

Chapter 3, a follow-up study on the Boeck-Bruusgaard material was carried out by Gjestland in 1955.[16] When Clark and Danbolt reviewed this material to provide a brief resume of the results of the study for the American literature, some of the results revealed that:

1. Untreated syphilitics exceeded the expected mortality rates by 53 percent in males and 63 percent in females.

2. Cardiovascular syphilis was observed to have developed in 13.6 percent of the males and 7.6 percent of the females. (Total: 9.7 percent.)

3. Neurosyphilis developed in 9.4 percent of the males and in 5.0 percent of the females. (Total: 6.5 percent.)

4. The mortality from syphilis among males was twice that of females.

5. Twenty-three percent had clinical or autopsy evidence of syphilitic pathology of a serious nature.[17]

A study on the outcome of untreated syphilis is being carried out by the United States Public Health Service. This is a continuing clinical study, including autopsy investigations. The study group consisted of male Negroes aged twenty-five and over and included 412 syphilitic males who had never received treatment, and 204 presumably nonsyphilitic Negro males as a control group. This study, well known as the "Tuskegee Study," began in 1932. Findings from this include the following:

1. After infections of fifteen years' duration, only one-fourth of the untreated syphilitics were normal, with most of the abnormal findings in the cardiovascular system.[18]

2. Mortality records during the first twelve years of observation revealed that 25 percent of the syphilitic and 14 percent of the controls of comparable ages had died. At age twenty-five, untreated male syphilitics would have a reduction of life expectancy of approximately 20 percent.[19]

3. After twenty years of follow-up, the life expectancy of individuals with syphilis from ages twenty-five to fifty was determined to be reduced by 17 percent. A Negro male with untreated syphilis of more than ten years' duration and a sustained reactive serology would have approximately a 50-50 chance of having demonstrable (autopsy information) cardiovascular involvement.[20]

Another study concerned with the outcome of untreated syphilitic infection was done by Rosahn at Yale.[21] He analyzed autopsy records from 1917 to 1941, consisting of 3,907 cases over the age of twenty. The results from this study indicated that:

1. Some 9.7 percent of the population studied had clinical, laboratory, or anatomic evidence of syphilis. This agreed with the results obtained in 1938 by Vonderlehr and Usilton, who estimated that in the United States a person stood one chance in ten of acquiring syphilis, before he died.[22]

2. Syphilitic males with lesions at autopsy comprised 4.7 percent of the male population, and syphilitic females with lesions constituted 2.7 percent of the female population. Sex appeared to exert a definite influence on resistance to the tissue changes of late syphilis, and this was independent of race.

3. Syphilitic infection significantly reduced longevity, regardless of whether or not tissue lesions resulted.

4. There was no greater frequency of anatomic lesions among syphilitic Negroes than among syphilitic whites. However, more whites with anatomic lesions died primarily as the result of their syphilis than did Negroes. Although the difference was not statistically significant, the findings were contrary to the generally accepted belief that syphilis runs a more fatal course among Negroes than among whites.

5. About 39 percent of the untreated syphilitic patients (Yale group) were found at autopsy to have anatomic evidence of syphilis, as compared with Bruusgaard's finding of 35 percent showing clinical or postmortem organic lesions of syphilis.

6. In the Yale series and in the Boeck-Bruusgaard material, an identical 23 percent of the untreated syphilis population died primarily as a result of syphilitic disease.

7. Rosahn observed that untreated syphilis apparently had both a case fatality rate and a spontaneous cure rate of about one in five.

8. There was a close parallel between the observations from the Yale study and those reported by Bruusgaard.

The prevention of late manifestations (disability and fatalities) of untreated syphilis is ample justification for the most strenuous efforts to provide prompt and adequate treatment of all cases.

INTERPRETATION OF SYPHILIS MORTALITY DATA

One of the brightest spots in the data for the evaluation of the effectiveness of venereal disease control has been the reduction of some of the more severe residual aftereffects, as manifested in death and disability. Reported mortality due to syphilis and its sequelae may be considered an inverse measure of the effectiveness of past casefinding methods and the effectiveness of medicines used in the treatment of cases that were brought to medical attention.

General Trends in Deaths from Syphilis and Its Sequelae

The trends of death rates in the death registration states since 1900 are characterized by large reductions in the death rates for infectious diseases and by increases in the death rates for diseases at older ages.

Since the turn of the century, mortality rates for tuberculosis, syphilis and its sequelae, typhoid fever, dysentery, diphtheria, whooping cough, meningococcal infections, acute poliomyelitis, and measles have all shown marked declines. Of this group of diseases, only syphilis and tuberculosis had rates of 1.0 or more per 100,000 in 1965.

In general the trend of syphilis mortality rates from 1900 to 1965 may be divided into three main time periods. The initial period, from 1900 to about 1923, is characterized by ineffective therapy and practically no preventive effort to control syphilis. From 1900 to 1917 the death rates per 100,000 population for syphilis and its sequelae increased from 12.0 to 19.1; within the few years from 1918 to 1922 they declined and increased again. The decline in syphilis mortality rates following 1917 is believed to be associated with the influenza epidemic of 1918. The influenza epidemic had its effect on many other unrelated causes simply because the influenza condition was classified as the primary cause of death. After World War I ended, interest and annual appropriations for venereal disease control dwindled. The first national public health effort to control syphilis ended.

The second time period, from 1923 to 1938, is one of little preventive control, but a period when therapy, depending upon its availability, was more widely applied. From 1922 to 1929, death rates declined slowly from 18.0 to 15.6. The rates remained almost level, between 15.0 and 16.2 per 100,000 population, from 1930 to 1939. Malaria therapy for general paralysis was introduced in this country about 1923. This and other types of fever therapy quickly gained acceptance and their use increased rapidly. The mortality death rates due to general paralysis declined sharply after 1925 and probably is largely responsible for the overall leveling off of the total syphilis mortality rates between 1923 and 1938. In the trend of total syphilis mortality the decline in mortality rates from general paralysis was partly counterbalanced when deaths from aneurysm (except of heart) were included with the total syphilis tabulations beginning in 1921.

In 1935 the passage of the Social Security Act enabled many states to institute some venereal disease control measures. Public interest in the problem and public health efforts toward control continued to grow. The growing awareness of the magnitude of the syphilis problem as a national health hazard resulted in the establishment of a National Venereal Disease Control Program in 1938. Furthermore, the increasing availability and application of syphilis therapy was beginning to make inroads on syphilis as a cause of death. The effects of widespread detection and treatment programs are reflected in the rapid and continued decline of general paralysis as a cause of death, starting about 1923, and for the decline of total syphilis as a cause of death, starting about 1938-1939. (See Figure 7.1 and Tables A.II.5 and 6.)

The last time period covers the years since 1939, the period of the National Venereal Disease Control Program. Within a year after the

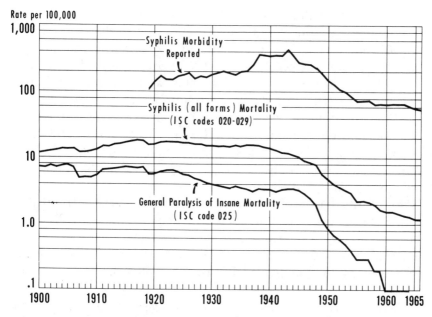

Fig. 7.1. Rates for syphilis mortality (1900 to 1965) and morbidity (1919 to 1965): United States.

program started, 1938 to 1939, activities were impressively increased as indicated by the following figures:

1. The number of new syphilis cases reported increased from 197,000 to 314,000, up 60 percent.

2. The number of diagnostic and treatment services in Venereal Disease Clinics increased from 4,767,000 to 6,864,500, up 49 percent.

3. The number of doses of arsenical drugs administered in Venereal Disease Clinics increased from 1,800,000 to 3,100,000, up 70 percent.

4. Doses of arsenical drugs distributed free to physicians increased from 2,700,000 to 4,600,000, up 67 percent.[23]

Between 1940 and 1945 millions of people were given blood tests for syphilis and treatment was administered when necessary. In 1943 penicillin was introduced into syphilis therapy. Early in the 1950's effective one-shot penicillin therapy for syphilis was being used. The dramatic effects of the widespread serologic screening dragnet, epidemiologic follow-up to find source and spread cases, plus the treatment of syphilis are reflected by the rapid and continued decline of syphilis as a cause of death starting about 1939.

In 1939 the death rate for syphilis was 15.0 per 100,000 population. By 1965 the death rate for syphilis had declined to 1.3 per 100,000 population. The death rate for syphilis was reduced more than 90 percent between 1939 and 1965. (See Tables A.II.5 and 6.)*

About 20,000 deaths due to syphilis were reported each year between 1933 (the year death-registration states became complete) and 1939. In 1939 deaths due to syphilis and its sequelae numbered 19,604 and were responsible for 1 out of every 71 deaths in the United States. By 1965 deaths due to syphilis numbered 2,434 and were responsible for only 1 out of every 751 deaths in the United States. (See Table A.II.5.)

Part of the decline in rates and numbers may be attributed to changes in the classification system, particularly the Sixth Revision, and the method for selection of the underlying cause of death. As discussed under "Classification of Deaths," 28 percent fewer deaths were assigned to syphilis and its sequelae when the cause of death

*Applying the comparability ratio to the syphilis mortality rates for 1939 would reduce the rate from 15.0 to 10.8 (15.0 x 0.72) per 100,000 population. This adjustment would not materially affect the interpretation of a great decline in syphilis mortality rates after 1939. Unless specified otherwise, the listed death rates refer to data tabulated by the revision of ISC in effect for the year in which deaths were reported.

was classified according to the Sixth Revision, beginning 1949, as compared with the same data classified according to the Fifth Revision. (See Table A.II.2.) However, the massive efforts to find cases (serologic screening procedures plus the epidemiologic efforts devoted to source and spread cases) and to treat large numbers of new and old cases of syphilis must be considered largely responsible for the reduction in the late manifestations of untreated syphilis and the continued decline of syphilis as a cause of death.

Syphilis Deaths by Age

The general pattern of syphilis mortality rates by age in 1910 was characterized by high infant mortality rates. Thus, in 1910 the death rate due to syphilis was very high during infancy (under one year of age), at 131.4 per 100,000; it dropped to a low of 0.4 at ages 5-14; thereafter it rose steadily with increasing age, reaching a peak rate of 47.5 at ages 75-84; and then the rate declined to 42.8 at ages 85 and over.

By 1939 the pattern of syphilis mortality rates by age was characterized by a lowered but still very high death rate among infants and a much higher death rate in ages 15-74. The highest death rates were still among infants under one year, 64.1 per 100,000, and 41.5 for ages 65-74. In 1965 the rate was only 0.6 per 100,000 among infants under one year of age; the peak rate was 9.2 at ages 75-84; and the death rates declined to 7.1 at ages 85 and over. Between 1939 and 1965 the largest relative declines in syphilis mortality rates took place in all age groups under 55, the most vigorous and productive part of life. (See Table A.II.6.)

Syphilis as a Cause of Death Among Infants Under One Year of Age

From the early part of the 1900's until the late 1930's the death rate from syphilis was relatively high in the first year of life when the disease is almost invariably congenital in origin.

In 1939 Dr. R. A. Vonderlehr estimated that each year 60,000 babies were born with syphilis, in addition to 25,000 still-births.[24] He also estimated that there were at least a million potential mothers in the United States infected with syphilis.

Syphilis deaths among infants under one year of age reached a high of 134.8 per 100,000 population during 1916 and then declined to a rate of 86.5 in 1923. From 1924 through 1937 the trend remained almost level, although the rates fluctuated between 77 and 87 per 100,000 population. (See Table A.II.6.)

Since the late 1930's there has been a sharp drop in the number of deaths from syphilis in children under one year of age. There were 1,300 deaths due to syphilis among infants under one year of age reported in 1939 compared to only 25 for this cause and age group reported during 1965. Syphilis deaths among infants under one year of age and the death rates per 100,000 live births are shown in Table A.II.7 for each state. During 1939 the death rate per 100,000 live births was highest in the West South Central States at 114.1 per 100,000 live births and lowest in the New England States at 15.8. In 1939 the syphilis death rate among infants under one year of age varied by state from a high of 217.0 per 100,000 live births in Louisiana to a low of 4.3 in Connecticut. In 1939 no infant deaths from syphilis were reported in Nevada or in Utah. (*Note*: In Table A.II.7 syphilis death rates are expressed as per 100,000 *live births.* All other death rates in other tables are expressed as per 100,000 *population.*)

In 1939, 1 out of every 84 deaths under one year of age was caused by syphilis; by 1965 only 1 in 3,715 deaths under one year of age was caused by syphilis. In 1939, 6.6 percent of the deaths certified as due to syphilis were in infants under one year of age; in 1965 it was only 1.0 percent.

As a cause of infant mortality, syphilis has practically disappeared. Many elements have contributed to this improvement. An important preventive measure was the legislation making blood tests mandatory before marriage and for pregnant women.

The decline in rates of infant mortality due to syphilis reflects not only improvement in venereal disease control efforts, but more specifically the prevention of congenital syphilis through treatment of syphilis in women during pregnancy and the finding and treating of children under one year of age who have congenital syphilis. Premarital testing also helped reduce infant syphilis deaths by detecting syphilis infections among marriage applicants. In spite of these preventive measures and other casefinding efforts, there were 3,505 cases of congenital syphilis reported in the United States during 1965; about 373 members of this group were children of one year of age or less. Prenatal or congenital syphilis can be totally prevented by frequent examinations, proper diagnosis, and adequate treatment of the infected mother. A greater effort must be made to provide the preventive measures necessary to eliminate syphilis completely as a cause of death and disease among infants under one year of age.

Syphilis Deaths by Sex and Color

Syphilis death rates have always been highest among the nonwhite males, second highest among nonwhite females, third highest among white males, and lowest among white females.

The highest rates for the white and nonwhite males and females occurred at different time periods. Syphilis death rates for white males reached a high of 24.0 per 100,000 population in 1917-1918; the rates for white females were highest during the years 1915-1917, at 10.1. The nonwhite male rate was highest in 1937-1938, at 77.6, and the highest rate observed for nonwhite females was 39.4 per 100,000 population in 1938. (See Table A.II.8.)

A comparison of the crude death rates indicates that the wide differential in syphilis mortality rates between the white and nonwhite groups, which existed during the late 1930's, has been reduced considerably. In 1939 the nonwhite syphilis death rate was 55.1 per 100,000 and this was 5.3 times higher than the white rate. In 1965 the nonwhite syphilis death rate was 2.8 per 100,000 and the rate differential between the nonwhite and white groups had apparently been reduced to about 2.5:1. (Table A.II.17.)

Age-Adjusted Syphilis Death Rates by Sex and Color

The reduction in the difference in syphilis mortality rates between the white and nonwhite groups which existed in 1939 may be more apparent than real. Death rates are affected by two important factors – the mortality prevailing at specific ages and the age distribution of the population for which they are computed. To facilitate comparisons, age-adjusted syphilis death rates by color and sex are presented in Table A.II.9. Any rate differences between these groups caused by different age distributions within the groups are removed by the adjustment process.

A summary of the age-adjusted syphilis death rates and differential ratios for 1939 and 1960 are presented in Table 7.1.

Table 7.1   Age-adjusted death rates for syphilis by color and
sex: United States, 1939 and 1959-61

Sex; color	1939	1959-61
	Age-adjusted rates	
Total	15.1	1.4
Male	21.5	2.2
Female	8.6	.7
White	10.3	1.0
Male	15.3	1.6
Female	5.2	.5
Nonwhite	62.5	5.3
Male	84.0	7.5
Female	40.0	3.4
	Ratio of nonwhite to white	
Total	6.1	5.3
Male	5.5	4.7
Female	7.7	6.8
	Ratio of male to female	
Total	2.5	3.1
White	2.9	3.2
Nonwhite	2.1	2.2

Sources: Vital Statistics Division, National Center for
Health Statistics: Vital Statistics - Special Reports, vol. 43,
no. 3, May 15, 1956, and special tabulations for 1959-61.

The results of adjusting the death rates by age show that the syphilis mortality differential between the white and nonwhite groups did improve a little between 1939 and 1960. However, the nonwhite rate is still 5.3 times higher than that of the white rate. The divergence between the age-adjusted death rates in 1960, for the two color groups is about 13 percent less than the 1939 level. Perhaps decreases in the syphilis death rate differentials were affected by casefinding and treatment efforts in the years preceding the decreases, and these efforts may have affected the nonwhite rates more than the white rates. The absolute magnitude of the decrease in syphilis death rates is much greater in the nonwhite rates since nonwhites had a much higher rate in 1939. Thus, while the age-adjusted syphilis death rates for the white group decreased a total of 9.3 per 100,000 population from 1939-1960, the nonwhite rate decreased by 57.2 per 100,000. (See Figure 7.2 and Table A.II.9.)

The age-adjusted death rate for nonwhite males was 5.5 times higher than the white male rate in 1939; this differential was lessened

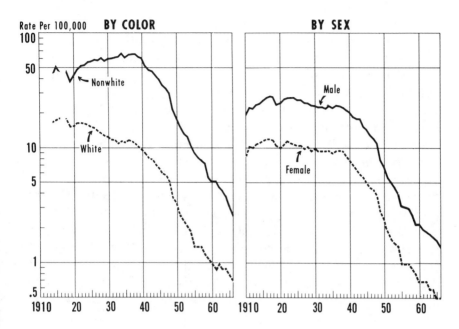

Fig. 7.2. Age-adjusted death rates for syphilis: (left) by color, United States, 1914-16, 1918-53, and 1960; (right) by sex, United States, 1910 to 1960.

to 4.7:1 in 1960. The age-adjusted death rate for nonwhite females was 7.7 times higher than the white female rate in 1939; this differential was somewhat lower at 6.8:1 in 1960.

In 1960 the white male age-adjusted rate was 3.2 times higher than the white female rate; this rate differential is slightly higher than it was in 1939. In 1960 the nonwhite male rate was 2.2 times higher than the nonwhite female rate; this is about the same rate differential observed for this color-sex group in the 1939 data. The overall male-female age-adjusted syphilis death rate differential increased from 2.5:1 in 1939 to 3.1:1 in 1960. (See Figure 7.2 and Table A.II.9.)

It is interesting to note that these relationships are quite different from those on reported syphilis case rates. For example, during 1960 reported syphilis case rates were approximately equal for males and females (1.3:1), although the age-adjusted death rate for males was much higher than for females.[25] The reported syphilis case rate for the nonwhite population was 10.9 times the rate for the white population, although comparison of reported age-adjusted death rates shows nonwhite rates to be 5.3 times the white rate.

These comparisons would suggest that among a group of syphilitics the risk of dying from syphilis may vary substantially by color and sex. However, in *Autopsy Studies in Syphilis,* Paul D. Rosahn concluded that the risk of dying from syphilis may vary with sex independent of race, but that the syphilis mortality rates between the white and nonwhite population might not be as widely separated as reported mortality rates indicate.

Some of the differences in white and nonwhite syphilis mortality rates may be due to a hesitancy of physicians in the reporting of syphilis as the cause of death among the white population. In the discussion concerning multiple conditions listed on the death certificate, it was noted that syphilis was listed somewhat more often as a contributory cause of death, rather than the primary cause, among the white than among the nonwhite population. This might tend to overemphasize the separation between the white-nonwhite syphilis death rates. However, the extent to which this factor affects the differential between white and nonwhite rates is not known. (See Table A.II.4.)

Parran stated that "Wherever education and living conditions among the Negro race approximate that of the white race, the syphilis rate approximates that of the white."[26] Clark and Danbolt, using the Boeck-Bruusgaard material, noted that "The mortality from syphilis among males was twice that of females. . ." [27] Both Moore[28] and Stokes[29] noted that syphilis was a milder disease in women than in men.

Rosahn made the following observations in a study of 3,907 autopsies performed in the Department of Pathology at the Yale University School of Medicine during the period 1917 to 1941:

1. There was no greater frequency of anatomic lesions among syphilitic nonwhites than among syphilitic whites.

2. Although more whites with anatomic lesions died primarily as the result of their syphilis than did nonwhites, the difference was not statistically significant.

3. Even in a group of women diagnosed as syphilitic on clinical, historical, or other evidence, syphilitic lesions occurred less frequently than in a comparable group of men. Therefore, sex appeared to exert a definite influence on resistance to the tissue changes of late syphilis, and this was independent of race.[30]

This information suggests that among a group of syphilitics the risk of dying from syphilis may indeed vary substantially by sex, independent of race. The results also appear to indicate that among a group of syphilitics the risk of dying from syphilis may not vary substantially between the white and nonwhite population.

The differentials in mortality between the white and nonwhite populations are the end-product of a multidimensional problem. Some of the factors that may affect this problem include the distribution and availability of medical facilities and services, socioeconomic factors which affect the utilization of available medical services, and the personal motivation to achieve better health.

Further study is needed to determine more accurately the degree that color and sex affect the risk of dying among a group of syphilitics.

Syphilis Deaths by Geographic Division and State

The national trend for syphilis deaths is paralleled by a similar trend in almost every geographic division and state. Analysis of syphilis mortality trends for individual states is limited to the examination of crude death rates because population estimates by age, sex, and color are not available annually on a consistent basis. The number of deaths and the crude death rates for syphilis are shown in Table A.II.10, for the United States, geographic divisions, and each state for selected years from 1933 to 1965.

In 1939 syphilis death rates were lowest in the New England States (9.9) and highest in the South Atlantic States (19.4). In 1965 there was little variation in the syphilis death rates among the geographic divisions, with all areas reporting rates less than or equal to 1.4 per 100,000 population.

In 1965 the crude death rate for syphilis was lowest in Tennessee (0.5) and highest in Wyoming (2.6). In 1939 the syphilis death rate was lowest in Utah (5.3) and highest in Florida (28.0).

Rate differences among states are more difficult to interpret than the trend lines within any state or for the nation. Factors affecting interstate comparison include the unknown amount of difference in reporting error which exists among different states, the prevalence of syphilis, the availability and utilization of treatment and medical facilities, mortality causes other than syphilis which may determine whether an infected person will live long enough to die of syphilis, the difficulty of diagnosing syphilis as a cause of death, and the willingness of physicians to report syphilis as a cause of death when they have made the diagnosis. The age, color, and sex variations in population from state to state may also affect the interstate syphilis death rate comparison. The extent that these factors do affect interstate rates is not known.

Syphilis deaths were tabulated by place of occurrence through 1941 and by place of residence beginning in 1942. This may have affected the trend data in some states. Between 1941 and 1942 particularly abrupt changes were evident in the crude death rates for syphilis in a number of states, including Alabama, Arizona, Arkansas, California, Florida, Louisiana, Missouri, Nevada, Oklahoma, South Carolina, Washington, and Wyoming.

Syphilis Deaths by Age for Geographic Division and State

Tables A.II.6 and 8 show deaths and death rates for syphilis by age, color, and sex for the United States in 1960. Summaries of the deaths and age-adjusted syphilis death rates by selected characteristics are presented in Tables A.II.8, 9, 11, and 13.

It is interesting to note that during the three year period 1959-1961 only 71 deaths from syphilis were reported among infants under one year of age. (See Table A.II.11). It was determined that some 56.3 percent of these infant deaths had occurred in the South Atlantic and West South Central States and that 26.8 percent of the infant deaths had occurred in the state of Texas.

In 1959-1961 the age-adjusted death rate for syphilis was highest (3.5 per 100,000 population) in the state of Louisiana. In general the higher age-adjusted syphilis death rates were recorded in the West South Central (2.0) and the South Atlantic States (1.8). (See Table A.II.13.)

The range of age-adjusted rates among geographic divisions in 1959-1961 was much smaller for the white population than for the nonwhite population. The following comparisons are made only for age-adjusted rates based on 20 or more deaths. The age-adjusted rates for white males was highest in the Pacific States (2.1) and in the West South Central States (2.0). The age-adjusted rates for white females was 0.7 or less in all of the geographic divisions. The age-adjusted rates for nonwhite males ranged up to 9.8 and 9.4 in the West South Central and West North Central States, respectively, while the rates for nonwhite females were highest in the Middle Atlantic (4.0) and in the West South Central States (3.9).

Within the geographic areas during 1959-1961 the age-adjusted syphilis death rate for the nonwhite population was generally higher than the rate for the white population. This rate differential was perhaps much lower in the Mountain and Pacific States because of the varying proportion of Negroes, American Indians, Chinese, and Japanese persons grouped under the nonwhite category.

As noted in another part of this chapter, among a group of syphilitics the risk of dying from syphilis may indeed vary substantially by sex, independent of color. However, among a group of syphilitics, the risk of dying from syphilis may not vary significantly between the white and nonwhite population.

The early detection and treatment of syphilis infections among females through serologic screening procedures such as prenatal testing would tend to prevent more syphilis deaths among them. This factor would also broaden the male-female rate differentials. Factors affecting the white-nonwhite rate differentials probably include economic status, degree of urbanization, the availability and utilization of medical services, and the personal motivations toward health.

The higher nonwhite rates and the rate differentials between the white and nonwhite populations throughout the nation may reflect the availability and utilization (or lack of utilization) of medical services or health programs by the population. Early treatment of syphilis infections prevents late manifestations. There is apparently little reason why the death rates from syphilis, especially among the nonwhite population, cannot be considerably reduced throughout the nation.

Syphilis Deaths for Urban and Rural Areas

In general syphilis mortality rates tend to be somewhat lower in rural areas than in urban areas. In 1959-1961 it was determined that some two-thirds of all syphilis deaths (64.4 percent for the white group and 70.9 percent for the nonwhite group) were among residents of metropolitan areas. The age-adjusted syphilis death rates in the metropolitan areas were higher than the rates noted in the nonmetropolitan areas for each of the color-sex groups. (See Table A.II.14.)

As far as the country as a whole is concerned, age-adjusted death rates for syphilis in the metropolitan countries of the southern states (South Atlantic, East South Central, and West South Central) tended to be higher than the rates observed in the nonmetropolitan areas.

This difference was more pronounced in the age-adjusted syphilis death rates for the nonwhite population. This may be due to a shift of population from the nonmetropolitan to the metropolitan areas. (See Table A.II.14.)

Syphilis Deaths by Marital Status

The relative risk of dying from syphilis varies considerably with marital status. It was determined that some 55.2 percent of all persons who died (all ages) from syphilis during the period 1959-1961 were married.

Using age-adjusted death rates, fifteen years and over for both males and females, married persons had lower syphilis death rates than the never married, widowed, or divorced groups. However, the differences are greater for males than for females.

For each color-sex group, the age-adjusted syphilis death rate for the divorced group was much higher than the married group. The divorced rate was the highest rate for white males, white females, and nonwhite males. The never married rate was the highest rate for nonwhite females. (See Table A.II.15.)

Although other factors may be present, the more favorable death rate from syphilis among the married population may be due to the premarital and prenatal screening tests for syphilis which detect syphilis infections early in life and thus prevent the damage of long-term untreated syphilis infections. Unfortunately, there are no routine screening procedures available for detecting syphilis infections early among the other groups.

Syphilis Deaths by Nativity of Population

During 1959-1961 it was determined that only 12 percent of the total syphilis deaths occurred among the white foreign-born population. All of the age-adjusted death rates for both white foreign-born males and females were based on a small number of deaths. (See Table A.II.16.) Adjusting the rates to eliminate differences in age distribution yields rates that are quite similar for the white foreign-born and for the white native-born population. Overall, the age-adjusted rate for the white foreign-born was only about 10 percent higher than the white native-born rate.

It was noted that in each geographic division where there were 140 or more syphilis deaths among the white foreign-born population, the age-adjusted death rate for the white foreign-born was somewhat lower than the age-adjusted rate for white native population. This was noted for the following geographic divisions: New England, Middle Atlantic, East North Central, and the Pacific. The other geographic divisions each had 68 or less syphilis deaths among the white foreign-born population, and the age-adjusted rates for the white foreign-born were somewhat higher than the age-adjusted rates among the white native-born population.

DETAILED CAUSE OF DEATH DUE TO SYPHILIS

The trend in total syphilis deaths and in death rates is a summation of a number of fatal syphilitic conditions. The various syphilitic conditions leading to death for 1940 and 1965 are listed in Table 7.2.

The relative importance of the fatal syphilitic conditions has changed over the years. Congenital syphilis, especially among infants under one year of age, has practically disappeared as a cause of death. While neurosyphilis accounted for 36.8 percent of the total syphilis deaths in 1940, it amounted to only 12.1 percent of the syphilis deaths in 1965. General paralysis of the insane, a form of

Table 7.2   Syphilis and its sequelae; number and percent of deaths by detailed cause: United States, 1940 and 1963

Detailed cause of death (ISC Code)	1940		1963	
	Number	Percent	Number	Percent
Syphilis and its sequelae (020-029)	19,006	100.0	2,666	100.0
Congenital syphilis (020)	1,290	6.8	31	1.2
Early syphilis (021)	---	---	---	---
Aneurysm of aorta (022)	3,635	19.1	1,441	54.0
Other cardiovascular syphilis (023)	1,525	8.0	767	28.8
Tabes dorsalis (024)	740	3.9	54	2.0
General paralysis of insane (025)	4,423	23.3	121	4.5
Other syphilis of the central nervous system (026)	1,819	9.6	191	7.2
Other syphilis (027-029)	5,574	29.3	61	2.3

Source: Vital Statistics Division, National Center for Health Statistics: Vital Statistics of the United States, 1940 and 1963.
    Note: Deaths tabulated according to revision of ISC in effect in the year in which deaths reported. ISC code numbers relate to seventh revision.

neurosyphilis, accounted for 23.3 percent of the total syphilis deaths in 1940, and only 3.9 percent during 1965.

Today syphilis of the heart and great blood vessels is the complication most likely to cause death. In 1940 deaths due to all cardiovascular syphilis (ISC Codes 022 and 023) accounted for only 27.1 percent of the total syphilis deaths; this cause accounted for 84.3 percent of the total syphilis deaths recorded during 1965. Summary data on deaths from syphilis by cause are shown in Tables A.II.5 and 18.

Cardiovascular Syphilis as a Cause of Death

Cardiovascular syphilis includes aneurysm of the aorta (ISC Code 022) and other cardiovascular syphilis (ISC Code 023).

Deaths from other cardiovascular syphilis (ISC Code 023) were tabulated separately beginning in 1939. In 1940 deaths from other cardiovascular syphilis numbered 1,525 with a rate of 1.2 per 100,000 population. The comparability ratios based on mortality statistics for the Fifth and Sixth Revisions increased the number of deaths from other cardiovascular syphilis 2.59 times. (See Table A.II.2) However, the numbers and rates continued to decline steadily and in 1965 there were only 549 deaths with a rate of 0.3 per 100,000 population from this cause. (See Table A.II.18.)

Aneurysm of the aorta (ISC Code 022) was designated as syphilitic beginning in 1939, and deaths from it were included with deaths from syphilis, except when the aneurysm was specified as non-syphilitic in origin, 1939-1954. Prior to 1939, aneurysm had little weight in the *Manual of Joint Causes of Death* and was frequently tabulated under associated causes. As a result of this change in classification, the reported death rate from syphilitic aneurysm of the aorta increased 50 percent, from a death rate of 2.0 in 1938 to 3.0 in 1939. (See Table A.II.5.) However, the death rates declined steadily after 1939. The comparability ratio for syphilitic deaths for aneurysm of the aorta between the Fifth and Sixth Revisions reduced deaths assigned to this cause by 46 percent. (See Table A.II.2). The number of deaths assigned to this cause was reduced further in 1955 by changes in the *Instruction Manual for Cause-of-Death Coding.*[31] Deaths from aneurysm of the aorta were included with deaths from syphilis in 1955 only if specified as syphilitic in origin.

Overall, deaths from aneurysm of the aorta decreased from 3,635 in 1940 to 1,504 in 1965, a death rate of 2.8 per 100,000 population and 0.8 in the respective years. However, the trend for the number of deaths from aneurysm of the aorta has been about level or increasing since 1955, the first year that deaths from aneurysm of the aorta were included with deaths from syphilis only if the physician specified the underlying cause of death as syphilitic in origin. In 1965 there were 1,504 deaths from aneurysm of the aorta compared to 1,337 in 1960 and 1,127 in 1955. The increases have been primarily in the white male and white female groups. Since 1960, deaths from this cause have remained fairly steady for the nonwhite group (See Tables A.II.5 and 18.)

The reasons for the recent increases in deaths from syphilitic aneurysm of the aorta are not apparent. Obviously, more deaths from aneurysm of the aorta are being specifically designated as syphilitic in origin by physicians. Also, scar tissue forms slowly and symptoms of inflammation of the aorta are difficult to recognize. Perhaps the increase in the number of deaths from this cause may be due to the difficulty of recognizing the symptoms in time for treatment to be of value.

Moore indicated that syphilis patients who develop aortitis with sacular aneurysm or aortitis with aortic regurgitation have an average duration of life of only one to three years following the onset of symptoms.[32] Kampmeier stated: "The prognosis in [syphilitic] aortic aneurysm is gloomy, death occurring commonly within a matter of months after the development of the symptoms and establishment of the diagnosis. A fair percentage of patients who are ill and are dying of syphilitic aortic insufficiency have negative serologic tests, whether of the flocculation or complement fixation variety."[33] Rosahn found in his autopsy studies that about one-fourth of all syphilitics with specific anatomic lesions had negative blood tests on the last admission to the hospital.[34]

The difficulty of diagnosis was also pointed out by Stokes as resulting from, "the silent invasion of the cardiovascular mechanism by *Spirochaeta pallida* and the latency ranging from several months to twenty-five or more years, when even the most thoroughgoing search fails to disclose a single abnormality. . . Paradoxically speaking, of the warnings, the first may be sudden death."[35]

Further reduction in the deaths from syphilitic aneurysm of the aorta will depend upon adequate early treatment. Kempmeier stated: "Treatment of the complications of syphilitic aortitis is prophylactic–the treatment of latent syphilis, and thus aortitis, before complications develop."[36]

Characteristics of Deaths from Cardiovascular Syphilis

It was determined that some 78.3 percent of the total syphilis deaths recorded during 1959-1961 were attributed to cardiovascular syphilis (ISC Codes 022-023). The majority (about 55 percent) of the total cardiovascular syphilis deaths were from syphilitic aneurysm of the aorta, ISC Code 022.

Some important differences were noted when deaths from syphilitic aneurysm of the aorta were compared with deaths from other cardiovascular syphilis. These differences have resulted from an increase over the past few years in the number of deaths from aneurysm of the aorta and a decrease in the number of deaths from other cardiovascular syphilis. Also, the nonwhite rates have generally been several times higher than the white rates for other cardiovascular deaths (ISC Code 023), whereas the nonwhite rates have been only about twice as high as the white rates for deaths caused by syphilitic aneurysm of the aorta. (See Table A.II.18.)

Since the number of deaths from cardiovascular syphilis make up such a large part (78 percent in 1960 and 84 percent in 1965) of the total syphilis deaths, the characteristics noted for total syphilis are heavily weighted by and therefore, similar to the characteristics of deaths caused by cardiovascular syphilis. With these considerations in mind, some of the characteristics of deaths caused by syphilis in the circulatory system, that is, total deaths from cardiovascular syphilis, including syphilitic aneurysm of the aorta may be noted.

Cardiovascular Syphilis Deaths by Age, Color, and Sex

Cardiovascular syphilis is generally not a cause of death in the very young age groups. Thus, during the three year period 1959-1961, cardiovascular syphilis caused no deaths among infants under five years of age and only 17 out of the total 6,946 deaths due to cardiovascular syphilis were under twenty-five years of age. About half of the male and female deaths from cardiovascular syphilis occurred among persons 65 years and over. However, cardiovascular syphilis deaths generally occurred at an earlier age in the nonwhite population than in the white population. For example, 39.8 percent of the cardiovascular syphilis deaths classed as white occurred among persons under 65 years of age while over 64 percent of the nonwhite deaths occurred in this age group. (See Table A.II.19.)

The cardiovascular syphilis mortality rates by age groups are considerably higher among the nonwhite population compared to the white population. The male death rates generally are two to three times higher than female rates.

For the country as a whole, the age-adjusted death rate, all ages, for cardiovascular syphilis was 1.1 per 100,000 population; ranging from a low of 0.4 noted among white females to a high of 5.8 noted among nonwhite males. Adjusting the rates for age differences tended to lower the rates for the white group and increase the rates for both nonwhite males and females.

Cardiovascular Syphilis Deaths by Geographic Division and State

Somewhat higher age-adjusted rates for cardiovascular syphilis deaths were recorded in the South Atlantic (1.4) and the West South Central States (1.6); with the lowest rate of 0.8 occurring in the East North Central States. (See Tables A.II.20 and 21.)

Excluding age-adjusted rates based on fewer than 20 deaths, the higher age-adjusted rates for white males were observed in the West South Central (1.6) and the Pacific States (1.8). The age-adjusted cardiovascular syphilis death rates for white females were 0.6 (Mountain States) or less in each geographic division.

The West South Central States had the highest nonwhite cardiovascular syphilis rates: 7.6 for nonwhite males and 3.2 for nonwhite females.

The age-adjusted cardiovascular syphilis death rate for the nonwhite population was generally about five times higher than the rate for the white population. As with total syphilis rates, the age-adjusted cardiovascular syphilis death rate differential, white to nonwhite, was somewhat lower in the Mountain and Pacific States – again, perhaps, due to the varying proportion of Negroes, American Indians, Chinese, and Japanese persons grouped under the nonwhite category.

Cardiovascular Syphilis Deaths for Urban and Rural Areas

For 1959-1961 it was determined that about 67.5 percent of all cardiovascular syphilis deaths (65.3 percent for the white group and 72.3 percent for the nonwhite group) were among residents of the metropolitan countries. The age-adjusted cardiovascular syphilis death rates were somewhat higher in the metropolitan, compared to the nonmetropolitan, areas for each color-sex group. (See Table A.II.22.)

Cardiovascular Syphilis Deaths by Marital Status

As with total syphilis deaths, the relative risk of dying from cardiovascular syphilis varies considerably with marital status. Some 58.2 percent of all deaths reported as cardiovascular syphilis, 1959-1961, were found to occur among married persons. Using age-adjusted rates, 15 years and over, the married group had the lowest rate while the divorced group had the highest rate. The age-adjusted rate for the divorced group tended to be two to three times higher than the rate for the married group and this was true for each of the color-sex groups, except the nonwhite female group, where the never married age-adjusted rate was slightly higher than the divorced rate. The rates for never married and widowed tended to fall between the rates found in the married and divorced groups. (See Table A.II.23.)

Cardiovascular Syphilis Deaths by Nativity of Population

During 1959-1961, it was determined that 12.7 percent (886) of the deaths from cardiovascular syphilis were among the white foreign-born population. Adjusting the rates for age differences yielded somewhat different rates for the white foreign-born and white native-born populations. (See Table A.II.24.) The age-adjusted rates may have a low degree of reliability due to the small number of deaths in these categories. Even so it was determined that the age-adjusted rate for the white foreign-born was some 12.5 percent higher than the age-adjusted rate for the white native-born population.

The cardiovascular syphilis deaths among the white foreign-born are largely in the older age groups. For example, it was determined that some 71.1 percent of the cardiovascular syphilis deaths are sixty-five years of age and over compared to 57.9 percent for the white native-born group. Much of the variance indicated here is due to the differences noted in the age distribution of the populations. Also, the excess of syphilis mortality among the white foreign-born may be due to the generally substandard living conditions of immigrants that existed in the early 1900's. Today, the new arrivals in this country benefit from improved surroundings, an improved standard of living, and better medical care. Perhaps this has helped reduce the acquisition of syphilis infections and the development of the late manifestations of untreated syphilis among the white foreign-born.

Neurosyphilis as a Cause of Death

The common types of neurosyphilis are tabes dorsalis, general paralysis of the insane, and meningovascular neurosyphilis. Symptomatic neurosyphilis is characterized by syphilitic damage to the central nervous system, resulting in neurologic, and often psychotic, signs and symptoms.

Tabes dorsalis (ISC Code 024), a diseased condition of the spinal cord, usually causing loss of control of the lower extremities (locomotor ataxia), develops more slowly than general paralysis and does not kill as early or as frequently as general paralysis. When death occurs it is usually due to some complicating disease or infection. The death rate from tabes dorsalis was 2.7 in 1910, 0.6 in 1940, and 0.0 in 1965. The number of deaths from this cause dropped from 740 in 1940 to 43 in 1965. (See Tables A.II.5 and 18.)

General Paralysis of the Insane as a Cause of Death

General paralysis of the Insane (ISC Code 025), often referred to as paresis, develops insidiously. Early signs are reflected in changes in personality and judgment. As the disease progresses the patient becomes gradually demented and bedridden. If untreated, the patient dies after two or three years.

The definition of general paralysis of the insane in the ISC has been fairly uniform over the entire period of national mortality statistics. Consequently, the trend of paresis death rates has been little affected by the periodic revisions of the ISC, with the possible exception of the Sixth Revision beginning in 1949. In the Sixth Revision, the number of deaths classified as due to general paralysis of the insane was reduced by 34 percent compared to the number so classified under the previous revision. (See Tables A.II.1 and 2.) If this adjustment were applied to the data, it would decrease the slope of the trend somewhat, but it would not materially affect the interpretation of a sharply declining trend of deaths due to general paralysis of the insane. Therefore, the data presented in this paper are based on deaths tabulated according to the revision of the ISC in effect in the year in which the deaths occurred.

Donohue and Remein divided the trend of general paralysis death rates into three time periods.[37] These periods are also generally applicable to the total syphilitic death trend. The initial period, from 1900 to 1923, a period of practically no preventive effort to control syphilis and of ineffective therapy, was characterized with almost level paresis mortality rates of 6.7 (geometric mean 1900-1923) deaths per 100,000 population. During the second time period, 1923 to 1938, malaria therapy and other types of fever therapy were introduced as treatments for general paralysis of the insane with a resultant decline in death rates. The third period covers the years 1938 to date, the period of the National Syphilis Control Program, a period of great preventive efforts to control syphilis. (See Figure 7.1 and Tables A.II.5 and 18.)

The death rate from general paralysis of the insane in the nonwhite population seemed resistant to control measures until about 1945-1946 when penicillin was introduced in the treatment of syphilis. After that period the considerable decline in deaths due to general paralysis was consistent for both white and nonwhite populations. In 1965 only 96 deaths were attributed to general paralysis of the insane. (See Table A.II.18.)

Without treatment, the ultimate clinical outcome in general paresis is usually death. Moore stated that with no treatment 80 percent of the paretics died within four years of onset.[38] The improvement in mortality rates over the years is striking. In a study of general paresis carried out by Malzberg, 78 percent of the male first admissions to mental hospitals with general paresis in 1910 died within five years after admission, compared to 47.2 percent in 1944-1949.[39] For females, the corresponding percentages were 62.5 and 38.9 respectively.

The mortality rates have also improved for all syphilitic psychoses. In a study by Kramer, it was noted that in 1914 some 41.2 percent of the syphilitic first admissions to mental hospitals died within the first year and that by 1948 this had been reduced to 20.6 percent.[40]

Fever therapy (introduced about 1923) was important in reducing the mortality from general paresis, but it was used primarily in treating patients who had already developed general paresis. The incidence of general paralysis continued to increase: "The rate of first admissions for paresis to State mental institutions increased from 4.1 in 1926 (the first year of the continuing census of mental institutions) to a peak of 5.1 per 100,000 population in 1939."[41]

Beginning in the late 1930's, the widespread treatment of syphilis cases undoubtedly prevented many cases from developing the late manifestations of untreated syphilis. In Figure 7.1 the decline in total deaths from syphilis and deaths from general paresis is graphically compared with the number of syphilis cases brought to treatment.

Neurosyphilis in Mental Hospitals

The preventive aspects of the syphilis control program are also evidenced through the reduction in the incidence of neurosyphilis in mental hospitals. First admissions to mental institutions for general paresis decreased from 7,261 in 1939 to 167 in 1965. In 1922 neurosyphilis was the cause of insanity in one out of every nine persons with psychoses admitted to mental institutions; by 1960, this had been reduced to about one out of every 164. The earlier detection of general paralysis plus more adequate treatment of patients with early syphilis has all but eliminated general paresis as a crippler and as a cause of death. (See Table A.II.25.)

Rates of first admissions to mental hospitals in the United States because of neurosyphilis fell from about 6.6 per 100,000 population in the late 1930's to 0.1 in 1965. By diagnosis, rates of first admissions to mental hospitals for general paresis and for other syphilitic involvements of the central nervous system were 5.5 and 1.0 per 100,000 population, respectively, in 1939 and 0.1 for both diagnoses combined in 1965. Correspondingly large decreases occurred in each state.

Although treatment for syphilitic psychoses enables many patients to return to their communities, some neurosyphilitic patients must be maintained (resident patients) in mental hospitals. The number of resident patients with syphilitic psychoses in mental hospitals declined from an estimated 42,000 during 1950 to an estimated 16,000 during 1965.[42] With the input (first admissions to mental hospitals with syphilitic psychoses) drastically reduced and decreasing, the number of resident patients with neurosyphilis should continue to decrease and, perhaps, approach zero in the future. However, the cost for maintenance of the resident patients with syphilitic psychoses in public mental hospitals was estimated at almost 45 million dollars for 1965. Obviously the dollar cost of not treating syphilis infections early is quite high.[43]

The future for neurosyphilis as a cause of insanity and death was summarized by Thomas: "Although all types of neurosyphilis can now be completely arrested or cured with penicillin, the goal we need to keep in mind is the prevention of symptomatic cases. This goal is on the way toward attainment and it should be attained in the near future if all medical facilities are alert in discovering syphilis before late symptoms develop."[44] He added a note of caution: "If paretics should increase in the future, [as a result of the increase of early infectious syphilis infections from 1957-1963] it will be a sad commentary on our casefinding methods because we usually have from 10 to 20 years to find and treat the syphilis before mental [and other] symptoms develop."

DEATHS CAUSED BY GONOCOCCAL INFECTION (ISC CODES 030-035)

While gonococcal infections cause blindness, temporary disability, and are a factor in the sterility of women, they have not been a significant cause of death. For example, in the United States deaths from gonococcal infections decreased from 419 in 1940 to 9 in 1965, a decrease of 98 percent. (See Table 7.3.)

Table 7.3   Deaths from gonococcal infection: United States, selected years (ISC codes 030-035)

| Color; sex | Number of deaths | | | |
	1940	1950	1960	1965
Total	419	37	38	9
Male	93	18	28	7
Female	326	19	10	2
White	200	8	12	3
Male	50	5	10	3
Female	150	3	2	-
Nonwhite	219	29	26	6
Male	43	13	18	4
Female	176	16	8	2

Source: "Comparability Ratios Based on Mortality Statistics for the Fifth and Sixth Revisions: United States, 1950." National Center for Health Statistics, Vital Statistics-Special Reports, vol. 51, no. 3, 1964.

Although gonorrhea has been almost eliminated as a cause of death and blindness, gonococcal infections still pose a major health problem. In the United States reported gonorrhea morbidity rose from 216,476 cases in 1957 to 310,155 cases in 1965, an increase of 43.3 percent.[45]

Gonorrhea control has been hampered by many factors including the number one priority assigned to the eradication of syphilis, the difficulty of diagnosing gonorrhea, particularly in the female, and the inadequacy of treatment resulting from the lessened susceptibility of the gonococcus to penicillin. However, during the syphilis eradication program increased emphasis has been placed on research devoted to gonorrhea. The smear and conventional culture, long the principal techniques for diagnosing gonorrhea, have been supplemented by the fluorescent antibody method for detecting the gonococcus and by the Thayer Martin VCN cultures medium which practically eliminates bacterial contamination of cultures. This latter contribution is of special value in diagnosing gonorrhea in the female since most specimens, particularly vaginal, are highly contaminated. The increasing resistance of the gonococcus to penicillin, which first became apparent in 1955, has been accompanied by a search for other antibiotics which may supplant penicillin when it has lost its effectiveness. Since resistance is not absolute, to date it has been counterbalanced by an adjustment upward of the amount of penicillin recommended for the treatment of gonorrhea.

These new advances and continuing research in the field of gonorrhea should be reflected in a decrease in the incidence of gonorrhea and a further reduction in the number of deaths from gonococcal infections.

BENEFITS DERIVED FROM THE PREVENTION AND CONTROL OF VENEREAL DISEASE

The prevention of the development of the late manifestations of syphilis has effected significant savings. Although it is not possible to estimate the total savings, some benefits can be determined by considering the savings in preventing deaths due to syphilis and the savings in preventing first admissions to mental institutions and in costs of hospitalization.

For example, if the color-sex syphilis death rates were still at the 1939 level, some 22,000 persons would have died from syphilis during 1965 instead of 2,434. (The expected number of deaths due to syphilis was adjusted downward according to the color-sex comparability ratios for the Fifth and Sixth Revision of the ISC. See Table A.II.2.) In other words, it is estimated that about 19,600 lives were saved from premature death in that one year (1965) as a result of the improvement in syphilis mortality conditions since 1939.

Similarly, if the rate of first admissions to mental institutions because of syphilitic psychoses was still at the 1939 level of 6.6 per 100,000 population, 13,000 persons with neurosyphilis would have been admitted to mental hospitals during 1965 instead of 232. The difference between these two figures represents the estimated admissions saved in just one year (1965), namely 12,800.

The median ages of reported syphilis deaths for selected years are shown in Table A.II.26. The median age of syphilis deaths has increased from 48.2 in 1933 to 68.1 in 1965. During this period the median age at death from all causes increased from 58.2 to 69.9. Apparently syphilis therapy has been quite effective in extending the years of life for persons who will die of syphilis. Also, the increasing median age may be an indication that the syphilis control efforts are effectively reducing the syphilis prevalence reservoir, thus preventing the development of the late and crippling manifestations of untreated syphilis. The decline in the late manifestations of untreated syphilis has had an incalculable effect on the health level of the nation.

In 1948 Kahn and Iskrant combined the effect of the lowered syphilis death rate and the increased age at death to compute the annual loss of life in years attributed to syphilis.[46] This calculation indicated that in 1933 white persons in the United States lost 290,303 years of life because of syphilis infection, and by 1944 the loss was reduced by 89,109 years. Complete data were not available to make a similar computation for nonwhite persons.

Venereal disease was once a major cause of blindness. Ophthalmia neonatorum, blindness in babies resulting from infection (usually with gonorrhea) by the mother during birth, was reported as causing 28.2 percent of the blindness in a sample group of children in schools for the blind in 1907. By 1954-1955 the percentage of ophthalmia neonatorum cases among new pupils entering schools for the blind had dropped to 0.1 percent.[47] This reduction was brought about largely through legislative measures that required the use of prophylactic drops in the eyes of newborn babies to prevent this disease.

During 1940 syphilis (interstitial keratitis) was responsible for an estimated 7.9 percent of all legal blindness in the United States. By 1957 the percentage was down to 3.8.[48] Syphilis as a cause of blindness for children of school age accounted for 5.2 percent of all cases in 1933-1934 and for 1.4 percent in 1954-1955. In 1954-1955 syphilis as a cause of blindness among new pupils accounted for only 0.6 percent of the total cases.[49]

The estimated prevalence of legal blindness caused by venereal disease was 28,100 in 1940 (18,200 caused by syphilis and 9,900 caused by ophthalmia neonatorum); by 1957 the estimated prevalence of blindness from this cause had been reduced to 14,600 (12,800 caused by syphilis and 1,800 caused by ophthalmia neonatorum).[50] Further reductions in the prevalence of blindness caused by venereal disease are expected in the future.

Preventive public health procedures combined with legislative backing have almost eliminated gonorrhea and syphilis as causes of blindness. Legislation requiring the use of prophylactic drops in the eyes of newborn babies was important in reducing the number blinded by gonorrhea. Legislation in many states requiring premarital and prenatal examinations for venereal diseases, especially syphilis, helped greatly in reducing syphilis infections as a cause of blindness and as a cause of death among infants.

Reducing the prevalence of blindness caused by venereal disease greatly reduces sociological and economic losses, both to the individual and to society. Benefits accrued through a reduction of blindness caused by venereal disease would include increased earning power for the individual, increased manpower for industry, a decrease in the cost for educating the blind, and a decrease in the economic aid for the blind. The extent of such benefits is unknown.

INTERNATIONAL: DEATHS CAUSED BY SYPHILIS IN SELECTED COUNTRIES

The number of deaths and the death rates for syphilis in selected countries, 1960 and 1965, are shown in Table A.II.27.

The United States is among the nations with the lowest death rates from syphilis. Nations having somewhat lower death rates include Australia, Bulgaria, Canada, Denmark, Greece, Israel, Mexico, Poland, and Sweden. Countries having somewhat higher rates include Czechoslavakia, England, Finland, France, Japan, Portugal, Spain, and Trinidad. The differences in syphilis death rates between countries might be greater if unreported deaths and age and sex differences in the populations could be taken into account. (See Table A.II.27.)

In 1951 Dublin estimated that there were more than 2,000,000 deaths from syphilis in the world annually.[51] In general, between 1952 and 1965, it was determined that most countries experienced a 50-60 percent decrease in the number of reported deaths from syphilis. Adjusting the estimated number of syphilis deaths in the world by the 50-60 percent decrease observed for reported deaths from syphilis would yield an estimated 800,000 to 1,000,000 deaths from syphilis in the world annually (1965).

In a study by Guthe it was noted that following 1954-1957 venereal syphilis showed a sustained rising incidence trend in all regions of the world.[52] This increase was noted in 76 out of 106 countries participating in the World Health Organization study. Further unfavorable developments must be expected unless the rising incidence trend is halted and syphilis infections treated early enough to prevent the complications of untreated syphilis. Syphilis is a worldwide problem, and it will take international planning and cooperation to eliminate it as a major health hazard throughout the world. The World Health Organization is already working in many areas to strengthen public health activities against syphilis.

SUMMARY

One of the objectives of syphilis control is to reduce the residual after-effects of untreated syphilis infections, as manifested in death and disability. Thus, the syphilis death rate has decreased from 15.0 per 100,000 population in 1939 to 1.3 in 1965. (Applying the Fifth-Sixth Revision comparability ratio would adjust the 1939 rate from 15.0 to 10.8.)

Even so, during 1965 there were 2,434 deaths attributed to syphilis and its sequelae. Some 84 percent of these deaths resulted from cardiovascular syphilis, primarily aneurysm of the aorta. The number of deaths from syphilitic aneurysm of the aorta has increased slightly during the last few years.

The reduction in the number of infant deaths caused by syphilis has been very impressive. While 1,300 infant deaths were caused by syphilis in 1939, the number of such deaths had been reduced to only 25 in 1965. However, there were 3,505 cases of congenital syphilis reported in the United States during 1965; about 373 members of this group were children of one year of age or less. A greater effort must be made to provide the preventive measures necessary to completely eliminate syphilis as a cause of death and disease among infants.

Deaths from syphilitic involvement of the central nervous system, especially general paralysis of the insane, was the main component of all syphilis deaths during the early part of the 1900's. In 1900 general paralysis accounted for 7.4 deaths per 100,000 population or about 60 percent of the total deaths due to syphilis and its sequelae. Although deaths from general paralysis started to decline after 1923 as soon as malaria (fever) therapy was introduced in the United States, the trend of deaths from this cause leveled off in the late 1930's. Following the nationwide venereal disease control efforts initiated in 1938 and 1939 and the introduction of penicillin therapy in the early 1940's, deaths from all types of syphilis, including general paralysis, began to decrease and there has been a constant downward trend ever since.

Neurosyphilis, especially general paresis of the insane, is no longer a major cause of admissions to mental institutions. In the early 1930's about one out of every ten admissions (psychoses) to mental institutions was due to neurosyphilis complications; by 1960 such admissions made up only six-tenths of one percent of the total. First admissions to mental institutions with general paralysis of the insane dropped from a rate of 5.5 per 100,000 population in 1939 to 0.1 in 1965.

Although the economic costs of uncontrolled syphilis have been greatly reduced since the early 1900's, they still remain needlessly high. For example, in 1965 the cost to the nation for maintenance of patients with syphilitic psychoses was estimated at nearly $45,000,000.[53]

The incidence and prevalence of blindness caused by syphilis and gonorrhea have been progressively decreasing. Even so, in 1957 the prevalence of legal blindness caused by venereal disease was estimated at 14,600 (12,800 caused by syphilis and 1,800 caused by ophthalmia neonatorum). Further reductions in the incidence and prevalence of blindness caused by venereal disease are expected in the future.

Further reduction of the late manifestations of untreated syphilis will depend upon the detection of the reservoir of unknown syphilis infections in the population. From the public health point of view, a large proportion of the reservoir must be found immediately after onset of the disease when the individuals are actually infectious. From the economic point of view, cases must be found before the late manifestations of untreated syphilis become evident through the destruction of blood vessels, nerve cells, or bones. Thus, to effectively prevent the spread of and to reduce the reservoir of unknown syphilis infections in the population there must be an epidemiological surveillance program designed to provide an early interception of source and spread infections. This procedure will greatly curtail the spread of syphilis infections in the community. Public education, designed to inform the public of the signs and symptoms of syphilis infections and to motivate persons infected with syphilis to seek medical attention immediately, will also help reduce the spread of syphilis in the community. In additon, there must be serologic screening programs to detect the reservoir of unknown syphilis infections for casefinding, leading to effective treatment, before the late manifestations of untreated syphilis occur.

The current methods of syphilis control combined with an available and effective therapy appear sufficient to completely eliminate syphilis as a crippler and as a cause of death in the United States. The elimination of syphilis requires adequate resources and personnel, the active support of the public, and the active cooperation and participation of the medical forces of the community. The degree to which these elements are present in a community's syphilis control program will determine how quickly syphilis will be eliminated.

These data are extremely encouraging and indicate that the late manifestations of untreated syphilis may eventually be practically eliminated. However, it is well to bear in mind this has not yet been accomplished and that every available resource must be mobilized to eliminate syphilis as a public health problem.

8 / Venereal Disease in the Military

Venereal disease among military personnel has been a serious problem from the era of the Greek city-states to the present time. In accounts of both field campaigns and peacetime activities, there is frequently some reference made to venereal infections and their adverse effect upon individual health and operational efficiency. In the past venereal disease has been rampant among the military forces of all nations, including those of the United States. Although case rates in this century have declined among the military, venereal diseases continue to be a problem among military forces in other nations and in the United States as well. Since most of the data under consideration are derived from Army figures, in this discussion the word "military" refers generally, but not exclusively, to Army personnel. However, infections among Naval forces are not uncommon and also constitute a problem.

Through the centuries various measures have been instituted by commanders to reduce the number of infections in their units. Punishment of individual soldiers for acquiring infection has long been an almost standard procedure and one which has been generally ineffective. Also ineffective has been the punishment of camp followers, who sometimes were punished by whipping, mutilation, or occasionally, death. A third technique, still in use in some countries today, has been to medically examine, treat, and license prostitutes around military installations. Although incidence has sometimes been temporarily reduced in this manner, the number of infections over a period of time usually remains high.

The most effective method of reducing incidence has been the introduction of different types of prophylaxis and education as to their use. Many countries, including the United States, instruct trainees in the use of prophylactic devices such as condoms, chemical preparations, and hygiene with soap and water. This approach has not eliminated infections but has generally been effective in reducing them. For example, in the American Army in World War I, it was made mandatory for members of certain units with high venereal disease rates to take prophylactic treatment after returning to their units from elsewhere, regardless of whether or not they admitted to sexual exposure. After this measure was instituted, two areas which previously had annual case rates of 625 per 1000 and 480 per 1000 (total venereal disease) dropped to 110 and 48, respectively.[1]

The extent of venereal disease among the military in past years has been discussed by Hinrichsen in *Venereal Disease in the Major Armies and Navies of the World.*[2] The causes for marked variation in rates between different armies or in one army at different times are not clear. The social and economic conditions within each country, the location of duty stations, the effects of war, and reporting procedures are some of the factors involved. In her study Hinrichsen does not compare the rates for different nations but uses them mainly to illustrate the extent of the problem.

Venereal Disease in the United States Army

The history of control measures for venereal disease in the United States Army dates to 1778 when the Continental Congress passed a bill making it possible to fine an infected individual for the cost of treating his disease. An Army regulation of 1814 provided that in addition to a fine, no soldier was to be in a pay status while under treatment for a venereal disease. Throughout the rest of the nineteenth century there apparently was little emphasis on venereal disease control. Gradually these infections emerged as a significant military health problem. At the turn of the century, the United States Army began to take a greater interest in the control and prevention of infection. Emphasis was placed on proper diagnosis and accurate reporting, a change which was reflected in a sudden increase in case rates starting in 1899. Prophylactic treatment after sexual exposure was introduced, and punishment for failure to report infections or employ prophylactic treatment was implemented in some areas.

In 1912 the War Department published an order providing for the confinement to post area and the withholding of pay of infected persons during the period of treatment. Unannounced physical examinations were used to detect unreported infections. The order of 1912 which provided for confinement and loss of pay also provided for the court martial of individuals who failed to take prophylactic treatment after exposure. Prophylaxis and punishment were to remain the mainstays of United States Army control programs almost until the end of World War II.

The punitive system was further refined in Europe during World War I. Court martial action was common not only for failure to employ prophylaxis but also for contracting infection, regardless of whether or not prophylactic treatment had been taken.

The seriousness of venereal diseases among United States military personnel is documented by medical records compiled during the war. In the American Expeditionary Force 3,500,000 total admissions to sick report were made. Of these admissions 358,000 or ten percent were for venereal infections. (The figures include all venereal diseases, acute and chronic, acquired either before or during active service.) Expressed as lost manpower, this meant that 18,000 men (one division) were out of action each day in 1918 because of venereal disease.[3] With a disease of such magnitude for which there was no totally effective cure but which could easily be prevented through sexual abstinence, it is understandable that military leaders should turn to punishment as a control measure.

By World War II some military men were suggesting that punishment, while partially effective in World War I, was not the answer to the problem.[4] The system was inherently unfair. Misconduct was allegedly being punished, but in reality, only the unlucky or careless were caught. Men who had illicit intercourse but did not acquire infection were no more or less virtuous than those who contracted disease. Men who took prophylactic treatment and still contracted a disease were treated no better than infected individuals who failed to take treatment. Persons treated in an on-duty status lost no pay or privileges, while those requiring hospitalization for treatment were denied pay during their stay in a hospital. Punishment fostered concealment, self-treatment, and inadequate treatment. Reduction in grade created a morale problem and reduced the overall efficiency of the Army during a period when manpower was critical. With the introduction of specific therapy in the form of penicillin, official punishment for venereal infections was abolished in 1944. Control programs since that time have been based on medical treatment and contact tracing.

United States Military Morbidity

Siler presented United States Army disease morbidity rates from 1820 to 1940.[5] This data is shown graphically in Figure 8.1.

Since present day diagnostic aids were not available during most of these years, Siler's figures represent clinical diagnoses and are subject to some degree of error. From Siler's tabular data, it is evident that syphilis and gonorrhea have been identified as different infections and classified as such by the United States Army since at least 1819.

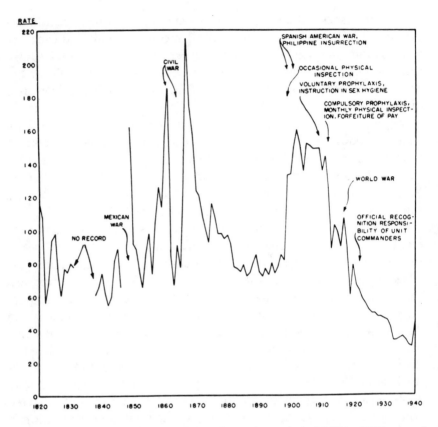

Fig. 8.1. Venereal disease in the United States Army from 1820 to 1940, annual rates per 100,000 strength.

Source: J. Siler, "The Prevention and Control of Venereal Diseases in the Army of the United States of America," *Army Medical Bulletin No. 67* (Pennsylvania, 1943).

This was sixty years before Neisser identified the gonococcus and nearly a century before *T. pallidum* was identified, indicating that although the etiologies of syphilis and gonorrhea were not fully understood, many nineteenth century physicians did in fact correctly consider them different infections.

Siler draws several conclusions from his data:

1. Venereal disease incidence is greatest during mobilization and in the initial stages of war.

2. Incidence drops when field campaigns are prolonged (Civil War, World War I), and remains stable or increases when campaigns are short (Spanish-American War, Philippine Insurrection).

3. Incidence increases after demobilization, with the highest rates in Army history occurring in 1867.

Table 8.1 illustrates military morbidity trends from 1947 through 1964. These figures were derived from published and special reports

Table 8.1   United States Military - Syphilis and gonorrhea case rates per 1,000 mean strength, personnel in the United States[a] and worldwide, 1947-64

Condition; fiscal year	Navy		Army		Air Force	
	World-wide	U.S.	World-wide	U.S.	World-wide	U.S.
Syphilis[b]						
1947	7.7	7.2	15.5	10.2	---	---
1948	6.6	5.5	12.9	5.7	---	---
1949	4.2	3.2	9.2	4.5	---	---
1950	2.4	1.7	6.4	3.2	4.1	2.2
1951	1.4	0.8	3.1	1.8	---	1.7
1952	0.7	0.5	2.8	1.9	---	1.4
1953	0.5	0.3	2.1	1.7	---	1.3
1954	0.4	0.2	1.6	1.0	1.2	1.0
1955	0.4	0.2	1.3	0.7	1.0	0.9
1956	0.3	0.2	1.4	0.8	1.0	0.9
1957	0.4	0.2	1.7	0.7	1.1	0.7
1958	0.4	0.3	1.5	0.6	0.8	0.4
1959	0.5	0.2	1.4	0.5	0.6	0.3
1960	0.5	0.2	1.2	0.5	0.6	0.2
1961	0.7	0.3	1.2	0.7	0.5	0.2
1962	0.8	0.3	1.2	0.7	0.5	0.3
1963	0.8	0.4	1.2	0.9	0.5	0.3
1964	0.8	0.4	1.5	0.9	0.5	0.3
Gonorrhea						
1947	80.3	52.8	83.8	54.0	---	---
1948	64.9	41.6	47.9	28.7	---	---
1949	45.6	25.2	41.2	20.8	---	---
1950	31.5	18.0	38.9	14.6	25.3	15.6
1951	37.1	14.1	31.2	18.1	---	12.0
1952	31.3	12.8	51.8	25.9	---	15.5
1953	31.8	15.4	54.3	28.8	---	19.0
1954	38.3	14.4	50.2	25.7	55.3	19.9
1955	46.2	14.1	50.5	22.3	56.2	19.8
1956	43.0	14.5	61.4	21.9	51.4	19.1
1957	42.5	14.6	49.8	22.0	50.1	18.8
1958	40.7	13.4	40.2	18.0	34.5	16.0
1959	45.1	11.4	37.0	15.8	34.5	14.5
1960	40.7	10.0	44.4	18.8	27.5	11.8
1961	39.1	10.6	49.9	23.9	20.9	10.3
1962	31.4	9.2	42.3	24.3	18.7	9.9
1963	29.6	10.1	43.6	24.7	19.4	10.5
1964	29.7	9.9	45.5	25.6	19.3	11.0

Source: Adapted from Statistics of Navy Medicine, Health of the Army, Monthly Medical Statistical Summary (Air Force) and special tabulations submitted to the Public Health Service by the Surgeons General of the Army, Navy, and Air Force.

[a] Army and Air Force excludes Alaska and Hawaii all years; Navy includes Alaska and Hawaii beginning 1960.

[b] Navy - early syphilis only; Army and Air Force - all stages of syphilis.

received by the Venereal Disease Program from the three military services.

Comparison of reported case rates of venereal disease among military personnel with civilian rates indicates considerably higher rates in the military than in the civilian population. This difference is probably due mainly to age bias, for the services are composed of young sexually active adults who would be expected on the basis of their age to have high case rates. Whether or not more complete reporting of diagnosed infections in the military accounts in part for the high rates is not known.

Comparison of rates of disease in the total military with personnel stationed in the United States indicates higher incidence rates among personnel stationed overseas. The trend of military rates for stateside personnel is generally consistent with the trend of United States civilian rates following World War II for both gonorrhea and syphilis. Both diseases showed large decreases from 1947 to the late 1950's after which there is some evidence of increased incidence of both syphilis and gonorrhea.

9 / International Venereal Disease Control

International programs for the control of infectious diseases have come into being only in the past century. They were originally promoted primarily by Western countries for the control of a few acute infectious diseases, but since their inception have been expanded to control many other diseases, and in practice include practically every nation in the world today. A major factor in the development of control measures was the promulgation and acceptance of Pasteur's germ theory of disease. Although the infectiousness of certain diseases has been recognized from the time of man's earliest civilizations, prior to the mid-nineteenth century, disease prevention as we practice it today was virtually unknown. Personal and environmental hygienic standards were low, and, as trade, travel, and emigration increased, the international spread of communicable diseases became more and more a matter of major concern. Pasteur's theory did not reduce the international or domestic transmission of infections overnight, but it did provide what proved to be a valid theory on which to base preventive measures.

In 1851 the First International Sanitary Conference was held, placing primary emphasis upon the prevention of infection through the use of quarantines, improvement of personal and environmental hygiene, and the alleviation of poverty and low standards of living. Control measures were directed toward the major virulent infections at that time—cholera, typhoid fever, typhus, smallpox, yellow fever, and plague.

By the end of the century the prevalence of these often fatal diseases had been reduced considerably, and the demonstrable success of control measures led to their increasing application. The general acceptance of international cooperation in disease control and prevention is illustrated by the establishment in 1907 of the *Office Internationale d'Hygiene Publique*, a permanent international health office. Cooperation between nations in matters of public health, though sometimes less than perfect, continues to this day.

When cholera, yellow fever, and other major pestilential diseases had been reduced to minor proportions, other less virulent, less infectious, but still highly prevalent diseases assumed greater prominence. Venereal diseases, particularly syphilis, were among the infections with new significance. The conferences which have been held concerning venereal disease control date to 1847, when the First International Conference on Venereal Disease was convened in Brussels. In this and subsequent conferences little could be done except to encourage the suppression of prostitution and traffic in women and discuss the broad social problems connected with venereal infections.

One of the major obstacles to venereal disease control was lack of effective therapy, for the preventive measures which were applicable to other diseases could not be employed for these infections. Further, sexual activity favoring transmission was apparently little influenced by lectures and admonitions on the danger of indiscriminate exposure. Fortunately, arsenotherapy was introduced in the treatment of syphilis in 1910, providing treatment which, while imperfect, often helped to reduce the further spread of infection even though the recipient himself was not adequately treated.

Further control measures, based both on prevention and treatment, were developed during and after World War I. The Health Organization of the League of Nations and the International Union against the Venereal Diseases contributed to improved methods of diagnosis, treatment, and control program operations. Probably the major accomplishment in international venereal disease control was the 1924 Brussels Agreement, a plan which provided medical care for merchant seamen and watermen. This agreement greatly facilitated treatment of infection and prevention of spread among a transient occupational group which had long been a major factor in venereal transmission. Although many nations, including the United States, were not signatories, provisions were subsequently made by most countries for the care of seamen in their ports and within their borders. In this country the 1938 La Follette-Bullwinkle Bill provided for care of merchant seamen in one of its provisions.

Since World War II, penicillin has significantly reduced the prevalence of infection among seamen, prostitutes, and other high incidence groups, and while international transmission of venereal disease still occurs, the problem in Western nations, at least, is small compared to past decades. In other nations, however, including many of those in Africa and Asia, prevalence and spread of venereal infections remain critical problems. Syphilis, gonorrhea, and the minor venereal diseases are undoubtedly far more widespread than the few reported cases indicate. Even greater problems in many of these nations are the treponematoses.

THE TREPONEMATOSES

Yaws, pinta, and endemic syphilis (bejel), the three treponematoses, are caused by pathogenic treponemes which are distributed by the blood and lymphatic systems and which in time become systemic, chronic, and destructive. Because they are usually contracted early in life, they are sometimes referred to as the endemic treponematoses of childhood. They are low-grade, herdtype infections, mild and chronic in their progression and less fatal in their results than syphilis or virulent infections such as smallpox and plague. Clinically their multiple manifestations are almost indistinguishable from those of venereal syphilis, and classification as separate diseases is based more upon ethnic and geographic occurrence than on microbiological characteristics. These diseases are found in areas where health is poor and sanitation primitive. They are found mainly in countries along or near the equator, and, while climate may be a factor in their transmission, the presence of endemic syphilis in parts of Europe in past centuries indicates that standards of living rather than geographical habitat is a significant consideration in their occurrence. As is true of the five venereal diseases, there is no known immunity to infection, but in areas where any one of these diseases is endemic, there is apparently strong resistance to infection from any other treponemal disease. Occurrence is mostly in childhood prior to puberty, but infection among adults is not unusual.

Yaws

A disease of the tropics and subtropics, yaws is found in equatorial Africa, Southeast Asia, the Caribbean, Central America, and northern South America.[1] It is an infection found only in man; males outnumber females in reported cases. Transmission is principally by direct, though not necessarily sexual, contact; infection *in utero* is not verified; indirect transmission is probably insignificant.

Yaws is also known as "frambesia," "bouba," "pian," and "parangi." The etiologic agent *Treponema pertenue* incubates for three to six weeks before symptoms appear. Manifestations are acute and chronic granulomatous and ulcerative lesions of the skin which can heal spontaneously and may later relapse. Cutaneous papules are the most common early symptom, and it is during this lesion period that infectiousness is greatest. Later, thickening and enlargement (hypertrophy) of the bones due to progressive destruction occurs. The central nervous system, eyes, and viscera are not known to be affected, and only rarely is the disease fatal. Darkfield examination, serologic tests, and clinical appearance are aids in diagnosis. Penicillin is the treatment of choice.

Pinta

Pinta is a nonvenereal infection caused by the *Treponema carateum.*[2] It occurs, like yaws in the tropics and subtropics, but mainly among dark-skinned peoples--Negroes, Indians, and persons of mixed blood. Pinta is geographically confined to the Western Hemisphere, principally to Mexico, Columbia, and Venezuela. The actual mode of transmission is unknown. What evidence is available suggests that the treponeme, identifiable in acute skin lesions, may be spread directly, indirectly, or even by vector agents. Little is known about congenital and venereal transmission.

After an incubation period of 7 to 20 days, a small primary chancre appears. This is shortly followed by pintids, erythematous cutaneous lesions similar to those of secondary syphilis. As the disease progresses, pigmented lesions develop, covering all or parts of the body with white, red, blue, pink, yellow, and violet splotches. From this pinta (Spanish "painted") acquires its name. Persons so afflicted are often referred to as *pintados.* Synonyms are "mal de pinto," "carate," "lota," or "spotted sickness."

In "painted" stages a good presumptive diagnosis can be made upon clinical appearance alone. Serologic tests are usually reactive. Penicillin is the preferred therapy.

Endemic Syphilis

Endemic syphilis (bejel or nonvenereal syphilis) is a treponemal infection which at one time was probably far more widespread than it is today.[3] Until recently, endemic syphilis prevailed in much of Western Europe (the "sibbens" of England and Scotland), and possibly was even present briefly in America among early colonists. Although the infection is no longer reported in Europe, it was prevalent as late as the mid-1950's in Bosnia, Yugoslavia.

Today endemic syphilis is localized in several scattered parts of the world, mostly in arid or semiarid countries. Incidence is most common in Africa (immediately north and south of the Sahara

Desert), the Eastern Mediterranean countries, Arab countries, central China, Turkey, and southern Russia. Different countries used names such as "radasyke," "njovera," "dichuhwa," and "sibbens" for the disease. Poor hygiene favors direct or indirect transmission from infectious skin lesions.

Like syphilis, bejel is caused by the *Treponema pallidum,* but the prognosis of bejel differs considerably from that of syphilis. After an incubation period of two weeks to three months, skin lesions resembling those of secondary syphilis appear, along with alopecia and mucous patches of the mouth. Primary lesions at the point of inoculation are almost never detected. After several years, destruction of the skin and long bones may occur, but central nervous system and cardiovascular involvement is uncommon; fatality is rare.

Diagnosis can be made on serologic tests and symptomatology. Penicillin is the treatment of choice.

Control Efforts

In 1948, when treponematoses eradication efforts were begun, it was estimated that 400,000,000 people lived in rural endemic treponematoses areas and that about 200,000,000 were actually infected. Guthe estimated that in the same year about 20,000,000 cases of venereal syphilis existed among persons 15 years of age or older, and that about 2,000,000 new infections occurred annually.[4] In addition to these there were a considerable, but undetermined number, of cases of venereally acquired gonorrhea. World Health Organization action was directed mainly against the treponematoses.

Since 1948, a mass penicillin treatment campaign has been conducted in many nations, mostly under the direction of the World Health Organization (WHO). Penicillin provides a cheap, quick, simple, and easily administered cure and has been tremendously effective in every area in which it has been used. Although WHO programs have not eradicated treponemal infections, these programs have relieved much suffering and returned to productivity many persons who would otherwise have been permanently incapacitated. In the two decades since treatment began, the reservoir of untreated cases has been lowered and new incidence decreased in many countries. In some few countries successful eradication has been achieved.

Three countries illustrate the effectiveness of the World Health Organization programs. In the early 1950's a project was undertaken to eradicate endemic syphilis in Bosnia, Yugoslavia; since 1957 no new cases have been reported. In Haiti a yaws eradication program was begun in 1950. Practically the entire island population received penicillin in a saturation treatment campaign. Transmission there has now ceased. In Western Samoa the prevalence of yaws was 11.3 percent in 1955. After a campaign less than 0.001 percent was found in 1958, and only isolated cases are now reported. These three countries illustrate the effectiveness of campaigns in small, isolated areas where control can be exercised to provide full coverage.

However, the geographic and socioeconomic circumstances of the countries in these examples are peculiar to them alone and, therefore, cannot be considered characteristic of all countries where the treponematoses are found. The results of programs in other countries, while encouraging, indicate that eradication is a long-term possibility which cannot be achieved while other socioeconomic factors are unchanged.

10 / Chancroid, Lymphogranuloma Venereum, and Granuloma Inguinale: The Three Minor Venereal Diseases

CHANCROID

Chancroid (also called soft chancre, soft sore, and chancre mou) is the most common of the minor venereal diseases in the United States. It is endemic in many parts of the world, particularly in tropical and subtropical countries. It is prevalent in all races, more common in urban than rural areas, and found more frequently in men than women. Although accidental infections among physicians and midwives have been recorded, transmission is almost exclusively by sexual intercourse. Indiscriminate promiscuity and poor personal hygiene favor transmission.

Chancroid is caused by *Hemophilus ducreyi,* or the bacillus of Ducrey. Found only in man, it is an organism to which there is no natural immunity. The normal incubation period is three to eight days; however, in damaged tissue, symptoms may appear twenty-four hours after infection. The lesion of chancroid is very similar in appearance to that of primary syphilis. It is manifested as an ulcerated sore at the point of inoculation and is later accompanied by swelling and suppuration of regional lymph nodes. Most lesions are located in the ano-genital area, but can appear anywhere on the body. Unlike chancres caused by syphilis, the lesions of chancroid are usually quite painful. Prognosis varies: some infections heal spontaneously; others progress rapidly, causing irreparable damage to the tissues involved. The period of infectiousness corresponds roughly to the duration of symptoms, but studies of the sex contacts of infected men suggest that asymptomatic women may be carriers.

Diagnosis can be based upon biopsy, autoinoculation, microscopic examination or culture. Darkfield and serologic examinations should be performed to exclude syphilis; lymphogranuloma venereum and granuloma inguinale should be excluded by specific tests.

Chancroid was first recognized as a separate disease in 1889 when Ducrey described the causative bacillus. It has been treated with topical applications of mercury and other heavy metals, washes, irrigations, powders, ointments, salves, caustics, and surgery, all to no avail. Surgery (such as circumcision) can even help the disease to spread by providing convenient openings in the skin. With the advent of sulfonamides, however, the first therapy specific for any of the venereal infections was discovered. Sulfa drugs are still the treatment of choice for chancroid, although streptomycin, aureomycin, or terramycin are also effective. These antibiotics should only be used after syphilis has been excluded as a possible concurrent infection. Sulfa preparations are particularly valuable as preferred treatment as their use will not mask syphilis symptoms or influence serologic reactivity.

LYMPHOGRANULOMA VENEREUM

Lymphogranuloma venereum is a venereally acquired infection attributed to a filterable agent of *lymphogranuloma venereum,* a bedsonia intermediate between bacteria and virus. It is characterized by genital lesions and inguinal lymphadenopathy. Synonyms include lymphogranuloma inguinale, climatic bubo, tropical bubo, lymphopathia venereum, and poradenitis venerea. The filterable agent causing the infection was discovered in 1931 by Hellerstrom and Wassen and can be microscopically detected with difficulty by skilled technicians. The disease is found only in man, but has been transferred experimentally to mice and ferrets.[1] Chick embryo is the best cultural medium.

There is apparently no natural or acquired immunity to infection. The incubation period is unknown; a few days to several months or even years may pass before symptoms appear. The length of time of communicability is also unknown and may vary from weeks to years. While lymphogranuloma venereum occurs throughout the world, it is most common in the tropics and subtropics. In the United States, it is diagnosed most frequently in the South and in large municipal areas. Males outnumber females in reported morbidity, but it is believed that both sexes are equally susceptible. Most cases occur among sexually active adults; however, cases among children are not uncommon. Because in many instances these children show no evidence of sexual abuse or intimate physical contact with adults, transmission through contaminated articles such as clothing is considered possible.

The first manifestation, often unnoticed, is a small erosion or papule at the point of inoculation. Within a few days a satellite bubo develops, accompanied by suppuration of regional lymph nodes, fever, chills, and headaches. At this time infection is most frequently detected. These symptoms may disappear through spontaneous healing in a few weeks, or may linger for several months before subsiding. The most common late symptoms are chronic adenitis in the male and elephantiasis in the female. Untreated, lymphogranuloma venereum remains chronic and destructive. The urogenital system in both sexes gradually deteriorates. Urethral damage may render urination difficult and cause retention of urine. Rectal strictures are particularly common in women and the resultant straining at defecation can cause utero-vaginal prolapse. In severe cases colostomy is necessary. In rare instances complications from infection may cause death.

As with chancroid, sufonamides have been the treatment of choice for lymphogranuloma venereum. Recently chlortetracycline and oxytetracycline have been used and show more promise than sulfa. Any of the broad spectrum antibiotics are beneficial. After the disease is cured, tissue or organ damage must be repaired surgically.

GRANULOMA INGUINALE

Although classified as a venereal disease, granuloma inguinale has never been proven to be transmitted sexually. It is presumably spread by direct contact during sexual intercourse; its almost exclusive manifestations in the ano-genital region support this theory. However, marital partners of infected persons are frequently free from disease, making the venereal mode of transmission questionable.

Granuloma inguinale (sometimes referred to as Donovaniasis, granuloma contagiosa, granuloma venereum, granuloma inguinale tropicum, ulcerating granuloma, and chronic venereal sore) is caused by *Donovanian granulomatis* (the Donovan body), an infection found only in man. The disease is found in all parts of the world, commonly among persons of low socioeconomic status, with incidence in both sexes variable. Racial and ethnic variations in reported cases are probably due to environmental factors and reporting practices.

The incubation period is unknown; estimates range from eight days to twelve weeks. The period of communicability is likewise unknown but is probably confined to the period of open lesions. Granuloma inguinale is a progressive infection of the skin and mucous membrane of the genitals and regional lymphatics. Extragenital infections occur occasionally in the mouth, on the lips, or between opposing skin surfaces. Many such infections are believed to result from autoinoculation after genital processes are fully entrenched. The first sign to appear is a vesicle, papule, or nodule. The surface epithelium becomes excoriated or eroded, leaving an ulcerated lesion with a beefy-red granular base. These usually appear on the glans or prepuce of the male, and on the labia, vagina, or cervix of the female. They are small and painless and consequently are frequently not detected in this stage. As the disease continues its insidious destructive progression, granulomatous ulceration of tissues and organs in the anogenital region occurs. Untreated infections can eventually cause marked impairment of health, anemia, debility, and sometimes death.

A highly accurate presumptive diagnosis of advanced cases can be made on clinical appearance alone.[2] Absolute diagnosis requires the demonstration of Donovan bodies in a spread of biopsy specimens. Granuloma inguinale was essentially incurable until the antibiotic era. At one time antimony preparations were used with limited success in early cases, but results were uncertain. Streptomycin, terramycin, aureomycin, and chloramphenicol are effective antibiotics, but definite cure is uncertain. Penicillin is not effective, but may be useful in treating accompanying infections and complica-search in this area is being conducted.

Appendices

Appendix I
Morbidity

The sources of all data in Tables A.I. are statistical summaries of reported cases of venereal disease submitted by the state departments of health to the Venereal Disease Branch of the Public Health Service.

Tables 1 through 3 present reported civilian venereal disease cases and rates by color and sex for the United States during fiscal years 1941-1966. Alaska and Hawaii are included in the United States totals beginning in 1958 and 1959, respectively. The District of Columbia did not report syphilis cases by stage of disease in fiscal year 1941 and is not included in the United States total for that year on Table 2. Rates for total cases are based on Bureau of the Census civilian population estimates as of January 1 (the midpoint) of each fiscal year. The color and sex specific rates are based on Bureau of the Census population estimates as of July 1 (the beginning) of each fiscal year. Prior to 1961, Connecticut did not report cases by color, and Connecticut cases were counted as white in arriving at the United States total cases, by color for the years 1941-1960.

In Tables 4 through 9, cases and rates of syphilis and gonorrhea are listed by state for selected fiscal years 1941-1966. State rates are based on Bureau of the Census estimates of the population as of July 1 of each fiscal year. Where no cases were reported, the tables indicate 0 cases and a rate of .0. Alaska and Hawaii are included in DHEW Region IX and United States totals beginning in fiscal year 1962.

Cases and rates of venereal disease for cities with more than 200,000 population for fiscal years 1957, 1962, 1965, and 1966 are presented in Tables 10 through 15. Rates are based on population estimates as of January 1 of each fiscal year by *Sales Management, Survey of Buying Power* (reproduction not licensed). Where no cases were reported, the tables indicate 0 cases and a rate of .0. Appropriate city or county populations were used for rate calculations for each reporting area. The use of city or county data is indicated by table footnotes.

Table 16 presents the age distribution of reported cases of congenital syphilis for the United States.

In Tables 17 and 18, the age distribution and rates of primary and secondary syphilis and gonorrhea are listed for the United States for the years 1956 and 1961-1965. Rates less than .05 are shown as 0.0.

Table A.I.1   Civilian cases and rates per 100,000 population for all stages of syphilis reported to the Public Health Service, by color and sex: fiscal years 1941-66

| Fiscal years | Number of cases | | | | | Rate per 100,000 population | | | | |
	Total	White Male	White Female	Nonwhite Male	Nonwhite Female	Total	White Male	White Female	Nonwhite Male	Nonwhite Female
1941	485,560	112,375	78,106	143,181	151,898	368.2	190.0	131.8	2,159.2	2,198.8
1942	479,601	111,492	70,492	155,766	141,851	363.4	190.7	117.7	2,342.6	2,024.1
1943	575,593	139,600	75,076	215,384	145,533	447.0	255.3	123.8	3,371.6	2,044.0
1944	467,755	101,542	70,430	160,587	135,196	367.9	193.9	114.8	2,576.3	1,868.8
1945	359,114	70,556	64,629	100,576	123,353	282.3	136.5	104.3	1,611.5	1,942.2
1946	363,647	80,274	62,264	103,197	117,912	271.7	141.1	99.1	1,542.5	1,576.7
1947	372,963	80,921	66,966	100,848	124,228	264.6	113.1	104.2	1,389.4	1,619.9
1948	338,141	70,139	57,060	94,123	116,819	234.7	110.2	87.5	1,256.5	1,489.1
1949	288,736	58,763	47,708	82,029	100,236	197.3	90.9	71.8	1,088.9	1,258.2
1950	229,723	45,570	38,081	65,644	80,428	154.2	69.4	56.5	855.2	993.4
1951	198,640	39,801	30,830	60,118	67,891	131.8	60.4	45.0	766.9	812.0
1952	168,734	34,584	27,565	50,031	56,554	110.8	52.4	39.5	631.7	659.9
1953	156,099	31,930	26,023	45,740	52,406	100.8	47.4	36.6	577.7	613.8
1954	137,876	28,787	22,998	40,305	45,786	87.5	42.0	31.8	497.2	523.4
1955	122,075	27,353	21,318	34,592	38,812	76.0	39.1	29.0	415.6	432.4
1956	126,219	27,325	21,194	37,393	40,307	77.1	38.3	28.3	437.2	438.6
1957	130,552	31,310	20,173	38,747	40,322	78.3	43.1	26.5	444.9	430.8
1958	116,630	26,085	18,701	35,563	36,281	68.5	35.3	24.1	392.9	373.8
1959	119,981	27,566	19,604	36,400	36,411	69.3	36.7	24.9	390.1	365.3
1960	120,249	29,843	20,654	35,718	34,034	68.0	39.1	25.8	371.1	334.0
1961	125,262	31,974	21,473	38,062	33,753	69.7	40.7	26.6	380.6	319.9
1962	124,188	31,798	21,310	37,176	33,904	68.1	40.0	26.0	367.5	314.9
1963	128,450	32,499	22,935	38,031	34,985	69.3	40.7	27.3	364.7	312.9
1964	118,247	29,454	20,561	35,837	32,395	62.9	36.5	24.1	338.0	284.0
1965	113,018	26,479	18,164	35,909	32,466	59.7	32.6	21.3	332.5	279.2
1966	110,128	24,239	17,030	36,696	32,163	57.1	29.3	19.5	243.9	270.2

Table A.I.2 Civilian cases and rates per 100,000 population according to stage of syphilis reported to the Public Health Service, by color and sex: selected fiscal years from 1941 to 1966

Fiscal year	Number of cases					Rate per 100,000 population				
	Total	White		Nonwhite		Total	White		Nonwhite	
		Male	Female	Male	Female		Male	Female	Male	Female
Primary and secondary syphilis										
1941	68,231	17,727	11,518	19,957	19,029	51.7	29.9	19.4	300.9	275.4
1947	106,539	27,836	18,611	31,559	28,533	75.6	44.8	29.1	437.3	374.2
1957	6,251	1,711	602	2,290	1,648	3.8	2.4	.8	26.3	17.6
1962	20,084	4,972	1,177	8,242	5,693	11.0	6.3	1.4	81.5	52.9
1965	23,250	4,213	1,358	10,138	7,541	12.3	5.2	1.6	93.9	64.8
1966	22,473	3,567	1,169	10,163	7,574	11.6	4.3	1.3	91.9	63.6
Early latent syphilis										
1941	109,018	16,292	14,431	35,009	43,286	82.6	27.5	24.3	527.9	626.6
1947	107,767	14,725	16,847	28,487	47,708	76.4	23.6	26.3	395.0	626.1
1957	19,046	3,938	2,656	5,230	7,222	11.4	5.4	3.5	60.1	77.2
1962	19,924	4,347	2,402	6,453	6,722	10.9	5.4	2.9	63.8	62.4
1965	17,315	3,179	1,516	6,343	6,277	9.1	3.9	1.8	58.7	54.0
1966	16,974	2,963	1,436	6,766	5,809	8.8	3.6	1.6	44.9	48.8
Late and late latent syphilis										
1941	202,984	55,499	33,509	57,123	56,853	153.9	93.8	56.5	861.4	823.1
1947	121,980	30,594	23,298	31,795	36,293	86.5	49.1	36.4	440.5	476.0
1957	96,856	24,171	14,859	29,164	28,662	58.1	33.3	19.5	334.9	306.2
1962	78,264	21,324	15,982	21,212	19,746	42.9	26.9	19.5	209.6	183.4
1965	67,636	18,133	13,860	18,445	17,198	35.7	22.3	16.2	170.8	147.9
1966	66,149	16,772	13,133	18,814	17,430	34.3	20.3	15.1	125.1	146.4
Congenital syphilis										
1941	17,600	4,121	4,647	3,904	4,928	13.4	6.9	7.8	58.8	71.3
1947	12,271	2,212	3,238	2,994	3,827	8.7	3.5	5.0	41.4	50.1
1957	5,452	719	1,378	1,335	2,020	3.3	1.0	1.8	15.3	21.6
1962	4,085	663	1,280	848	1,294	2.2	.8	1.6	8.4	12.0
1965	3,505	575	1,072	709	1,149	1.9	.7	1.3	6.6	9.9
1966	3,464	589	957	756	1,162	1.8	.7	1.1	5.0	9.8

Table A.I.3 Civilian cases and rates per 100,000 population for gonorrhea reported to the Public Health Service, by color and sex: fiscal years 1941-66

| Fiscal years | Number of cases | | | | | Rate per 100,000 population | | | | |
| | Total | White | | Nonwhite | | Total | White | | Nonwhite | |
		Male	Female	Male	Female		Male	Female	Male	Female
1941	193,468	86,647	30,986	51,435	24,400	146.7	146.5	52.3	775.6	353.2
1942	212,403	77,768	33,020	76,313	25,302	160.9	133.0	55.1	1,147.7	361.0
1943	275,070	85,325	46,090	97,701	45,954	213.6	156.0	76.0	1,529.4	645.4
1944	300,676	95,707	61,882	92,044	51,043	236.5	182.7	100.9	1,476.7	705.5
1945	287,181	74,109	75,114	76,299	61,659	225.8	143.4	121.2	1,222.5	970.8
1946	368,020	98,103	72,900	123,728	73,289	275.0	172.4	116.1	1,849.4	980.0
1947	400,639	94,437	53,190	170,556	82,456	284.2	157.1	81.3	2,340.6	1,070.1
1948	363,014	82,588	40,975	171,359	68,092	252.0	129.7	62.9	2,287.8	868.0
1949	331,661	68,249	33,703	165,235	64,474	226.7	105.5	50.8	2,193.2	809.3
1950	303,992	51,834	26,952	163,065	62,141	204.0	78.8	39.9	2,100.0	759.1
1951	270,459	43,298	20,258	149,235	57,668	179.5	65.7	29.5	1,903.5	689.9
1952	245,633	36,857	18,809	130,829	59,138	161.3	55.8	27.0	1,648.1	688.8
1953	243,857	35,430	17,635	127,419	63,373	157.4	52.6	24.8	1,609.2	742.2
1954	239,661	34,824	15,337	129,513	59,987	152.0	50.8	21.2	1,597.7	685.8
1955	239,787	34,440	14,737	129,678	60,932	149.2	49.3	20.0	1,557.9	678.8
1956	233,333	33,742	13,570	126,709	59,312	142.4	47.3	18.1	1,481.6	645.4
1957	216,476	30,958	12,626	119,700	53,192	129.8	42.7	16.6	1,374.4	568.3
1958	220,191	31,346	13,014	121,128	54,703	129.3	42.4	16.8	1,338.1	563.7
1959	237,318	36,168	15,064	128,194	57,892	137.1	48.1	19.1	1,373.7	580.8
1960	246,697	42,574	16,132	132,050	55,941	139.6	55.7	20.2	1,371.8	549.0
1961	265,665	48,398	19,220	140,023	58,024	147.8	61.6	23.8	1,400.2	549.9
1962	260,468	50,107	19,368	139,052	51,941	142.8	63.1	23.6	1,374.4	482.5
1963	270,076	55,329	20,025	143,960	50,762	145.7	69.3	23.9	1,380.4	454.0
1964	290,603	59,056	22,224	158,577	50,746	154.5	73.1	26.1	1,495.6	444.8
1965	310,155	62,201	23,854	171,023	53,077	163.8	76.6	27.8	1,583.7	456.4
1966	334,949	67,561	26,547	185,831	55,010	173.6	81.8	30.4	1,235.6	462.1

Table A.I.4 Civilian cases and rates per 100,000 population for all stages of syphilis reported to the Public Health Service by state and territorial health departments: selected fiscal years from 1941 to 1966 (known military cases excluded)

States by DHEW Regions	1941 Cases	1941 Rate	1947 Cases	1947 Rate	1957 Cases	1957 Rate	1962 Cases	1962 Rate	1965 Cases	1965 Rate	1966 Cases	1966 Rate
Connecticut	2,027	118.4	2,163	114.5	880	39.6	761	29.2	689	25.2	644	22.8
Maine	718	84.8	901	107.1	47	5.9	65	6.7	184	18.9	279	28.6
Massachusetts	4,550	105.2	3,789	85.6	1,949	40.9	2,609	50.3	1,982	37.4	1,787	33.6
New Hampshire	308	62.5	360	73.8	148	26.7	101	16.5	100	15.5	79	11.9
Rhode Island	1,124	158.3	1,096	148.1	483	60.7	309	36.6	400	45.2	348	38.9
Vermont	174	48.6	277	81.2	51	13.9	10	2.5	12	2.9	21	5.3
Region I	8,901	105.4	8,586	98.4	3,558	37.1	3,855	36.3	3,367	30.6	3,158	28.6
Delaware	1,543	577.9	1,003	336.6	1,001	254.1	802	178.2	753	156.2	517	104.0
New Jersey	10,568	253.9	9,670	223.0	5,020	93.7	5,596	90.2	5,311	80.1	3,943	58.5
New York	43,052	320.2	33,524	247.7	19,857	123.0	22,647	135.5	19,879	111.2	18,866	104.7
Pennsylvania	18,216	183.4	17,412	178.5	3,318	30.3	10,765	95.3	5,690	49.7	4,961	43.1
Region II	73,379	263.9	61,609	220.7	29,196	88.9	39,810	114.8	31,633	86.8	28,237	77.0
Dist. of Col.	8,391	1,239.4	4,245	477.0	1,957	232.6	1,927	260.1	1,728	217.7	1,473	186.7
Kentucky	6,930	244.1	6,527	244.1	1,911	64.0	1,726	56.9	1,706	54.7	1,723	54.8
Maryland	10,887	595.9	7,670	347.1	2,405	87.7	2,845	90.8	3,142	93.0	3,243	93.7
North Carolina	18,167	565.2	9,034	251.6	4,498	103.8	3,829	84.5	2,282	47.9	2,242	46.5
Virginia	18,438	687.5	11,153	363.2	3,648	104.5	3,327	84.8	2,475	58.5	1,972	45.9
West Virginia	7,700	403.4	8,593	469.6	1,514	76.4	1,307	70.7	1,081	60.2	1,436	79.2
Region III	72,513	537.1	47,222	331.0	15,933	97.3	14,961	86.9	12,414	68.7	12,089	66.0
Alabama	21,616	763.3	19,257	668.0	1,410	45.3	1,538	46.9	2,207	65.3	1,928	56.1
Florida	20,216	1,057.3	17,963	758.3	7,315	199.0	5,986	116.5	5,530	98.7	6,320	110.6
Georgia	20,960	674.8	11,974	373.0	3,945	108.5	3,549	90.6	2,479	59.0	2,526	59.2
Mississippi	50,224	2,310.2	17,946	898.6	1,351	64.2	571	26.1	841	36.7	951	41.3
South Carolina	18,562	982.6	8,028	429.8	6,963	302.4	2,418	102.6	1,765	70.9	1,742	70.0
Tennessee	19,603	668.6	11,817	387.1	1,798	52.2	1,894	52.7	1,947	51.6	1,389	36.4
Region IV	151,181	1,018.4	86,985	565.6	22,783	124.7	15,956	77.9	14,769	68.0	14,856	67.5
Illinois	22,131	280.6	21,320	264.4	5,713	61.0	7,800	77.7	6,135	58.8	7,188	67.8
Indiana	6,766	197.7	7,057	194.1	1,697	38.5	1,364	29.0	1,192	24.7	1,075	22.0
Michigan	9,824	186.0	17,226	294.4	4,784	63.8	3,476	43.8	5,346	66.3	5,784	70.7
Ohio	20,411	294.9	16,643	222.9	7,578	83.5	3,378	34.3	4,717	46.8	4,277	41.9
Wisconsin	1,216	38.7	2,383	76.1	1,324	35.2	744	18.5	969	23.6	1,368	33.1
Region V	60,348	226.4	64,629	229.6	21,096	61.8	16,762	45.9	18,359	49.0	19,692	51.8

Iowa	2,603	103.1	1,717	72.1	1,302	48.4	923	33.2	823	29.8	851	30.9
Kansas	2,908	163.1	2,656	154.0	1,422	69.0	1,124	52.1	867	39.6	977	44.5
Minnesota	2,546	91.5	1,636	60.4	187	5.8	255	7.4	230	6.5	204	5.8
Missouri	10,874	287.4	10,036	271.0	4,705	111.4	4,265	98.0	4,238	96.9	3,503	78.4
Nebraska	960	73.4	2,216	181.5	378	27.0	436	30.8	413	28.2	373	25.6
North Dakota	393	61.7	328	60.6	36	5.5	28	4.4	21	3.4	19	3.1
South Dakota	586	92.0	539	97.6	165	24.0	142	20.7	201	28.4	115	16.5
Region VI	20,870	154.6	19,128	149.1	8,195	54.8	7,173	46.3	6,793	43.4	6,042	38.3
Arkansas	11,259	579.5	10,430	594.3	2,736	152.6	1,647	92.1	1,087	56.7	1,257	64.5
Louisiana	10,199	431.6	14,593	580.7	6,465	218.3	5,080	153.8	2,924	85.2	2,869	81.8
New Mexico	1,450	271.5	1,507	276.0	1,541	194.8	1,085	112.8	515	52.2	942	93.5
Oklahoma	8,501	368.6	7,699	362.5	1,386	62.9	1,541	66.2	1,430	58.8	1,204	49.3
Texas	31,355	490.1	15,786	225.6	3,572	40.9	4,676	48.6	5,205	50.9	5,528	53.2
Region VII	62,764	463.4	50,015	358.9	15,700	95.2	14,029	78.0	11,161	58.8	11,800	61.2
Colorado	3,865	342.0	2,042	177.4	504	32.3	542	30.9	599	31.1	509	26.4
Idaho	354	67.6	787	155.2	99	15.9	27	4.0	17	2.5	17	2.4
Montana	338	60.8	489	99.0	309	48.8	224	33.2	188	27.1	145	20.8
Utah	908	164.5	460	72.2	232	28.7	164	18.0	160	16.1	139	14.1
Wyoming	499	202.8	363	141.8	72	23.3	19	5.7	70	20.8	101	30.2
Region VIII	5,964	198.3	4,141	136.0	1,216	30.9	976	22.4	1,034	22.2	911	19.7
Alaska	207	279.7	127	158.8	23	14.3	47	23.4	32	14.7	32	14.6
Arizona	2,018	397.2	1,475	230.1	2,145	207.3	840	61.3	689	43.9	561	35.4
California	22,883	330.1	25,058	257.9	9,146	72.2	8,544	53.1	11,634	65.5	11,726	64.1
Hawaii	865	217.3	802	167.1	117	22.2	87	14.6	108	16.9	130	20.1
Nevada	375	331.9	600	419.6	142	59.4	180	62.1	316	79.0	231	53.5
Oregon	1,433	130.3	1,536	110.2	658	38.4	530	29.6	354	19.0	362	19.2
Washington	2,931	169.9	1,979	88.0	484	18.7	438	15.4	358	12.2	251	8.6
Region IX	29,640	285.6	30,648	216.7	12,875	69.0	10,666	46.0	13,488	53.2	13,293	51.1
United States	485,560	368.2	372,963	264.6	130,552	78.3	113,522	68.1	113,018	59.7	110,128	57.1
Puerto Rico	—	—	7,759	365.1	1,560	69.2	1,078	46.1	1,578	61.5	2,197	83.6
Virgin Islands	—	—	132	488.9	145	604.2	257	803.1	483	1,380.0	528	1,508.6
Canal Zone	—	—	312	650.0	113	289.7	60	171.4	119	340.1	131	374.3
U.S. & Terr.	486,632	368.0	382,095	265.8	132,510	78.0	114,917	68.0	115,198	60.0	112,984	57.7

Note: Alaska and Hawaii included in U.S. & Territories total for fiscal years 1941, 1947, and 1957 and in DHEW Region IX and United States totals beginning with fiscal year 1962.

Table A.I.5 Civilian cases and rates per 100,000 population for primary and secondary syphilis reported to the Public Health Service by state and territorial health departments: selected fiscal years from 1941 to 1966 (known military cases excluded)

States by DHEW Regions	1941		1947		1957		1962		1965		1966	
	Cases	Rate	Cases	Rate	Cases	Rate	Cases	Rate	Cases	Rate	Cases	Rate
Connecticut	196	11.4	436	23.1	61	2.8	126	4.8	150	5.5	103	3.7
Maine	202	23.8	483	57.4	9	1.0	11	1.1	7	0.7	4	0.4
Massachusetts	553	12.8	1,212	27.4	232	4.9	398	7.7	263	5.0	331	6.2
New Hampshire	21	4.3	100	20.5	4	0.7	11	1.8	23	3.6	14	2.1
Rhode Island	99	13.9	252	34.1	3	0.4	28	3.3	20	2.3	31	3.5
Vermont	56	15.6	161	47.2	4	1.1	3	0.8	1	0.2	2	0.5
Region I	1,127	13.3	2,644	30.3	313	3.3	577	5.4	464	4.2	485	4.4
Delaware	121	45.3	364	122.1	23	5.8	39	8.7	70	14.5	46	9.3
New Jersey	1,143	27.5	2,019	46.6	113	2.4	991	16.0	1,040	15.7	828	12.3
New York	3,408	25.3	7,367	54.4	703	4.4	3,876	23.2	3,464	19.4	3,329	18.5
Pennsylvania	1,986	20.0	4,386	45.0	129	1.2	923	8.2	475	4.2	567	4.9
Region II	6,658	23.9	14,136	50.6	968	3.0	5,829	16.8	5,049	13.9	4,770	13.0
Dist. of Col.	—	—	1,579	177.4	106	12.6	702	94.7	551	69.4	468	59.3
Kentucky	1,095	38.6	2,683	100.3	43	1.4	166	5.5	187	6.0	125	4.0
Maryland	1,204	65.9	2,379	107.6	235	8.6	561	17.9	466	13.8	555	16.0
North Carolina	3,319	93.0	4,404	122.6	216	5.0	620	13.7	1,082	22.7	976	20.2
Virginia	4,088	152.4	3,808	124.0	158	4.5	400	10.2	339	8.0	296	6.9
West Virginia	1,226	64.2	3,689	201.6	21	1.1	51	2.8	71	4.0	100	5.5
Region III	10,932	81.0	18,542	130.0	779	4.8	2,500	14.5	2,696	14.9	2,520	13.8
Alabama	2,788	98.4	3,272	113.5	149	4.8	562	17.1	1,306	38.6	1,252	36.4
Florida	3,217	168.3	4,126	174.2	173	4.7	1,356	26.4	2,168	38.7	2,103	36.8
Georgia	1,178	37.9	3,789	118.0	555	15.3	946	24.1	1,067	25.4	1,014	23.8
Mississippi	6,588	303.0	7,207	360.9	66	3.1	106	4.8	519	22.7	647	28.1
South Carolina	6,270	331.9	2,608	139.6	508	22.1	707	30.0	845	33.9	882	35.5
Tennessee	3,109	106.0	4,033	132.1	201	5.8	345	9.6	564	15.0	342	9.0
Region IV	23,150	155.9	25,035	162.8	1,652	9.0	4,022	19.6	6,469	29.8	6,240	28.3
Illinois	2,088	26.5	6,044	74.9	464	5.0	1,002	10.0	1,356	13.0	1,260	11.9
Indiana	1,286	37.6	2,117	58.2	60	1.4	86	1.8	72	1.5	76	1.6
Michigan	1,303	24.7	3,924	67.1	118	1.6	294	3.7	732	9.1	1,057	12.9
Ohio	2,698	39.0	4,925	66.0	168	1.9	281	2.9	637	6.3	623	6.1
Wisconsin	240	7.6	670	21.4	58	1.5	52	1.3	84	2.0	89	2.1
Region V	7,615	28.6	17,680	62.8	868	2.5	1,715	4.7	2,881	7.7	3,105	8.2

Iowa	434	17.2	650	27.3	15	0.6	20	0.7	33	1.2	72	2.6
Kansas	604	33.9	762	44.2	24	1.2	54	2.5	19	0.9	62	2.8
Minnesota	207	7.4	623	23.0	20	0.6	83	2.4	108	3.1	56	1.6
Missouri	1,702	45.0	3,131	84.6	79	1.9	190	4.4	267	6.1	214	4.8
Nebraska	241	18.4	465	38.1	4	0.3	11	0.8	63	4.3	78	5.3
North Dakota	91	14.3	159	29.4	-	-	3	0.5	1	0.2	5	0.8
South Dakota	155	24.3	198	35.9	8	1.2	20	2.9	55	7.8	36	5.2
Region VI	3,434	25.5	5,988	46.7	150	1.0	381	2.5	546	3.5	523	3.3
Arkansas	1,836	94.5	2,821	160.7	63	3.5	249	13.9	244	12.7	152	7.8
Louisiana	2,116	89.5	4,680	186.2	90	3.0	1,294	39.2	737	21.5	649	18.5
New Mexico	330	61.8	537	98.4	35	4.4	67	7.0	122	12.4	101	10.0
Oklahoma	1,162	50.4	1,626	76.6	44	2.0	113	4.9	140	5.8	110	4.5
Texas	4,124	64.5	3,430	49.0	541	6.2	1,415	14.7	1,378	13.5	1,544	14.9
Region VII	9,568	70.6	13,094	94.0	773	4.7	3,138	17.4	2,621	13.8	2,556	13.2
Colorado	990	87.6	723	62.8	35	2.2	59	3.4	38	2.0	59	3.1
Idaho	123	23.5	230	45.2	31	5.0	2	0.3	6	0.9	9	1.3
Montana	80	14.4	177	35.8	16	2.5	3	0.4	24	3.5	35	5.0
Utah	139	25.2	128	20.1	23	2.8	4	0.4	16	1.6	18	1.8
Wyoming	142	57.7	143	55.9	8	2.6	1	0.3	3	0.9	7	2.1
Region VIII	1,474	49.0	1,401	46.0	113	2.9	69	1.6	87	1.9	128	2.8
Alaska	67	90.5	65	81.3	3	1.9	6	3.0	7	3.2	7	3.2
Arizona	309	60.8	638	99.5	58	5.6	124	9.0	280	17.9	201	12.7
California	3,085	44.5	6,070	62.5	494	3.8	1,572	9.8	1,939	10.9	1,768	9.7
Hawaii	109	27.4	79	16.5	1	0.2	12	2.0	21	3.3	35	5.4
Nevada	24	21.4	176	123.1	20	8.4	50	17.2	56	14.0	32	7.4
Oregon	334	30.4	511	36.7	32	1.9	40	2.2	54	2.7	55	2.9
Washington	521	30.2	624	27.8	31	1.2	49	1.7	80	2.7	48	1.6
Region IX	4,273	41.2	8,019	56.7	635	3.4	1,853	8.0	2,437	9.6	2,146	8.3
United States	68,231	51.7	106,539	75.6	6,251	3.8	20,084	11.0	23,250	12.3	22,473	11.6
Puerto Rico	-	-	952	44.8	57	2.5	395	16.9	840	32.7	982	37.4
Virgin Islands	-	-	23	85.2	1	4.2	36	112.5	24	68.6	30	85.7
Canal Zone	-	-	58	120.8	10	25.6	25	71.4	37	105.7	37	105.7
U.S. & Terr.	68,407	51.7	107,716	74.9	6,323	3.7	20,540	11.1	24,151	12.6	23,522	12.0

Note: Alaska and Hawaii included in U.S. & Territories total for fiscal years 1941, 1947, and 1957 and in DHEW Region IX and United States totals beginning with fiscal year 1962.

Table A.I.6 Civilian cases and rates per 100,000 population for early latent syphilis reported to the Public Health Service by state and territorial health departments: selected fiscal years from 1941 to 1966 (known military cases excluded)

States by DHEW Regions	1941		1947		1957		1962		1965		1966	
	Cases	Rate	Cases	Rate	Cases	Rate	Cases	Rate	Cases	Rate	Cases	Rate
Connecticut	133	7.8	489	25.9	195	8.8	217	8.3	153	5.6	142	5.0
Maine	46	5.4	108	12.8	5	0.6	5	0.5	9	0.9	7	0.7
Massachusetts	—	—	547	12.4	252	5.3	307	5.9	271	5.1	296	5.6
New Hampshire	17	3.4	56	11.5	16	2.9	4	0.7	15	2.3	6	0.9
Rhode Island	138	19.4	129	17.4	25	3.1	30	3.6	20	2.3	32	3.6
Vermont	50	14.0	29	8.5	2	0.5	—	—	—	—	3	0.8
Region I	384	9.3	1,358	15.6	495	5.2	563	5.3	468	4.3	486	4.4
Delaware	235	88.0	345	115.8	141	35.8	40	8.9	38	7.9	25	5.0
New Jersey	2,161	51.9	3,426	79.0	511	9.5	760	12.3	972	14.7	574	8.5
New York	5,396	40.1	7,384	54.6	1,749	10.8	4,202	25.1	4,457	24.9	4,326	24.0
Pennsylvania	5,608	56.5	5,932	60.8	540	4.9	1,041	9.2	335	2.9	278	2.4
Region II	13,400	48.2	17,087	61.2	2,941	9.0	6,043	17.4	5,802	15.9	5,203	14.2
District of Columbia	—	—	1,508	169.4	298	35.4	329	44.4	363	45.7	327	41.4
Kentucky	897	31.6	1,660	62.1	92	3.1	50	1.6	59	1.9	61	1.9
Maryland	420	23.0	1,634	73.9	225	8.2	435	13.9	407	12.0	470	13.6
North Carolina	8,457	237.0	3,116	86.8	878	20.3	661	14.6	303	6.4	345	7.2
Virginia	4,795	178.8	4,074	132.7	642	18.4	237	6.0	170	4.0	195	4.5
West Virginia	1,001	52.4	2,275	124.3	118	6.0	65	3.5	24	1.3	35	1.9
Region III	15,570	121.4	14,267	100.0	2,253	13.8	1,777	10.3	1,326	7.3	1,433	7.8
Alabama	6,046	213.5	5,075	176.0	394	12.7	605	18.4	616	18.2	401	11.7
Florida	3,403	178.0	6,287	265.4	1,276	34.7	1,869	36.4	997	17.8	1,012	17.7
Georgia	13,063	438.8	3,838	119.6	932	25.6	754	19.2	492	11.7	549	12.9
Mississippi	11,926	548.6	5,424	271.6	140	6.7	87	4.0	182	7.9	116	5.0
South Carolina	4,668	247.1	3,547	189.9	1,425	61.9	471	20.0	333	13.4	386	15.5
Tennessee	5,946	202.8	4,400	144.1	278	8.1	195	5.4	228	6.0	162	4.2
Region IV	45,052	303.5	28,571	185.8	4,445	24.3	3,981	19.4	2,848	13.1	2,626	11.9
Illinois	4,283	54.3	6,398	79.3	1,053	11.2	1,607	16.0	1,157	11.1	1,305	12.3
Indiana	539	15.8	1,280	35.2	191	4.3	204	4.3	146	3.0	167	3.4
Michigan	1,498	28.4	3,993	68.2	974	13.0	227	2.9	298	3.7	522	6.4
Ohio	3,578	51.7	4,981	66.7	1,273	14.0	430	4.4	525	5.2	558	5.5
Wisconsin	68	2.2	520	16.6	136	3.6	68	1.7	114	2.8	111	2.7

Iowa	653	25.9	478	20.1	72	2.7	12	0.4	13	0.5	21	0.8
Kansas	376	21.1	637	36.9	63	3.1	58	2.7	42	1.9	40	1.8
Minnesota	234	8.4	244	9.0	21	0.7	29	0.8	22	0.6	41	1.2
Missouri	3,907	103.3	3,154	85.2	416	9.9	396	9.1	265	6.1	183	4.1
Nebraska	185	14.1	523	42.8	12	0.9	27	1.9	22	1.5	26	1.8
North Dakota	62	9.7	51	9.4	2	0.3	6	0.9	2	0.3	1	0.2
South Dakota	127	19.9	159	28.8	39	5.7	8	1.2	30	4.2	26	3.7
Region VI	5,544	41.2	5,246	40.9	625	4.2	536	3.5	396	2.5	338	2.1
Arkansas	3,073	158.2	4,062	231.5	206	11.5	101	5.6	74	3.9	55	2.8
Louisiana	329	13.9	3,599	143.2	632	21.3	687	20.8	477	13.9	411	11.7
New Mexico	191	35.8	445	81.5	209	26.4	107	11.1	86	8.7	101	10.0
Oklahoma	1,824	79.1	1,928	90.8	171	7.8	112	4.8	68	2.8	97	4.0
Texas	7,454	116.5	4,977	71.1	868	9.9	1,264	13.1	1,155	11.3	1,240	11.9
Region VII	12,871	95.0	15,011	107.7	2,086	12.7	2,271	12.6	1,860	9.8	1,904	9.9
Colorado	251	22.2	520	45.2	97	6.2	48	2.7	50	2.6	46	2.4
Idaho	1	–	206	40.6	20	3.2	9	1.3	2	0.3	1	0.1
Montana	1	0.2	97	19.6	24	3.8	16	2.4	24	3.5	13	1.9
Utah	81	14.7	95	14.9	16	2.0	32	3.5	24	2.4	17	1.7
Wyoming	48	19.5	81	31.6	7	2.3	3	0.9	3	0.9	2	0.6
Region VIII	381	12.7	999	32.8	164	4.2	108	2.5	103	2.2	79	1.7
Alaska	6	8.1	39	48.8	9	5.6	10	5.0	3	1.4	6	2.7
Arizona	222	43.7	382	59.6	435	42.0	180	13.1	122	7.8	106	6.7
California	4,847	69.9	6,976	71.8	1,798	13.7	1,780	11.1	2,050	11.5	2,029	11.1
Hawaii	36	9.0	112	23.3	16	3.0	20	3.4	9	1.4	11	1.7
Nevada	85	75.9	3	2.1	27	11.3	28	9.7	24	6.0	19	4.4
Oregon	268	24.7	234	16.8	93	5.4	29	1.6	11	0.6	30	1.6
Washington	428	24.8	461	20.5	57	2.2	62	2.2	53	1.8	41	1.4
Region IX	5,850	56.4	8,056	57.0	2,410	12.9	2,109	9.1	2,272	9.0	2,242	8.6
United States	109,018	82.7	107,767	76.4	19,046	11.4	19,924	10.9	17,315	9.1	16,974	8.8
Puerto Rico	–	–	3,426	161.2	372	16.5	443	18.9	484	18.9	657	25.0
Virgin Islands	–	–	87	322.2	36	150.0	108	337.5	222	634.3	217	620.0
Canal Zone	–	–	83	172.9	13	33.3	21	60.0	43	122.9	49	140.0
U.S. & Terr.	109,060	82.4	111,514	77.6	19,492	11.5	20,496	11.1	18,064	9.4	17,897	9.1

Note: Alaska and Hawaii included in U.S. & Territories total for fiscal years 1941, 1947, and 1957 and in DHEW Region IX and United States totals beginning with fiscal year 1962.

Table A.I.7 Civilian cases and rates per 100,000 population for late and late latent syphilis reported to the Public Health Service by state and territorial health departments: selected fiscal years from 1941 to 1966 (known military cases excluded)

States by DHEW Regions	1941		1947		1957		1962		1965		1966	
	Cases	Rate	Cases	Rate	Cases	Rate	Cases	Rate	Cases	Rate	Cases	Rate
Connecticut	1,206	70.4	924	48.9	555	25.0	394	15.1	384	14.0	385	13.6
Maine	384	45.3	257	30.6	33	3.7	44	4.5	136	14.0	230	23.6
Massachusetts	3,694	85.4	1,819	41.1	1,328	27.9	1,639	31.6	1,273	24.0	1,021	19.2
New Hampshire	172	34.9	162	33.2	120	21.7	83	13.6	59	9.1	49	7.4
Rhode Island	750	105.6	503	68.0	346	43.5	180	21.3	204	23.0	162	18.1
Vermont	53	14.8	53	15.5	41	11.2	7	1.8	9	2.2	14	3.5
Region I	6,259	74.1	3,718	42.6	2,423	25.2	2,347	22.1	2,065	18.8	1,861	16.8
Delaware	215	80.5	172	57.7	745	189.1	633	140.7	527	109.3	361	72.6
New Jersey	5,880	141.2	3,936	90.8	4,207	78.5	3,650	58.9	3,111	46.9	2,412	35.8
New York	30,634	227.8	17,450	128.9	16,983	105.2	14,275	85.3	11,677	65.3	10,902	60.5
Pennsylvania	6,714	67.6	5,705	58.5	2,551	23.3	8,482	75.1	4,660	40.7	3,975	34.6
Region II	43,443	156.2	27,263	97.6	24,486	74.6	27,040	78.0	19,975	54.8	17,650	48.0
District of Columbia	----	----	970	109.0	1,515	179.7	857	115.7	709	89.3	638	80.9
Kentucky	2,501	88.1	1,497	56.0	1,593	53.4	1,256	41.4	1,115	35.8	1,247	39.7
Maryland	2,176	119.1	2,018	91.3	1,773	64.7	1,675	53.5	2,151	63.7	2,107	60.9
North Carolina	7,353	206.1	1,122	31.2	3,124	72.1	2,392	52.8	845	17.7	828	17.2
Virginia	7,891	294.2	2,828	92.1	2,457	70.4	2,335	59.5	1,651	39.1	1,324	30.8
West Virginia	1,427	74.8	2,319	126.7	1,215	12.4	1,159	62.7	944	52.6	1,244	68.7
Region III	21,348	166.5	10,754	75.4	11,677	71.3	9,674	56.2	7,415	41.4	7,388	40.3
Alabama	5,360	189.3	6,285	218.0	591	19.0	344	10.5	253	7.5	242	7.0
Florida	7,864	411.3	5,044	212.9	5,561	151.2	2,594	50.5	2,198	39.2	3,011	52.7
Georgia	6,314	203.3	3,900	121.5	1,865	51.3	1,702	43.3	879	20.9	908	21.3
Mississippi	13,868	637.9	4,386	219.6	1,051	50.0	347	15.8	115	5.0	172	7.5
South Carolina	6,596	349.2	1,655	88.6	4,483	194.7	1,133	48.1	512	20.6	381	15.3
Tennessee	9,485	322.5	3,036	99.4	1,202	34.9	1,300	36.1	1,109	29.4	850	22.3
Region IV	49,487	333.4	24,306	158.0	14,753	80.7	7,420	36.2	5,066	23.3	5,564	25.3
Illinois	14,900	188.9	8,306	103.0	3,897	41.6	4,879	48.6	3,448	33.0	4,378	41.3
Indiana	2,635	77.0	2,514	69.2	1,333	30.3	984	20.9	910	18.9	787	16.1
Michigan	4,691	88.8	6,548	111.9	2,604	34.7	2,327	29.3	3,894	48.2	3,727	45.5
Ohio	10,534	152.2	6,159	82.5	5,819	64.1	2,528	25.6	3,343	33.2	2,871	28.1
Wisconsin	871	27.7	1,042	33.3	835	22.2	532	13.2	703	17.1	1,022	24.7
		126.2		87.3	17,488	62.5	11,250	30.8	12,298	32.8	12,785	33.6

Iowa	1,209	47.9	437	18.3	1,099	40.9	813	29.3	712	25.8	701	25.4
Kansas	1,018	57.1	1,058	61.3	1,261	61.2	912	42.2	735	33.6	825	37.6
Minnesota	1,991	71.5	664	24.5	142	4.4	127	3.7	92	2.6	102	2.9
Missouri	4,297	113.6	3,173	85.7	4,038	95.6	3,483	80.1	3,459	79.1	2,384	64.5
Nebraska	494	37.8	772	63.2	324	23.1	371	26.2	306	20.9	242	16.6
North Dakota	123	19.3	71	13.1	31	4.7	19	3.0	17	2.7	12	1.9
South Dakota	239	37.5	156	28.3	102	14.8	107	15.6	104	14.7	51	7.3
Region VI	9,371	69.6	6,331	49.3	6,997	46.8	5,832	37.7	5,425	34.7	4,817	30.6
Arkansas	4,226	217.5	3,048	173.7	2,285	127.4	1,188	66.4	718	37.4	994	51.0
Louisiana	446	18.9	2,507	99.8	5,379	181.6	2,904	87.9	1,596	46.5	1,684	48.1
New Mexico	795	148.9	434	79.5	1,264	159.8	837	87.0	290	29.4	699	69.4
Oklahoma	2,631	114.1	3,004	141.4	1,078	48.9	1,227	52.7	1,160	47.7	930	38.0
Texas	12,086	188.9	2,099	30.0	1,968	22.5	1,507	15.7	2,454	24.0	2,577	24.8
Region VII	20,184	149.0	11,092	79.6	11,974	72.6	7,663	42.6	6,218	32.7	6,884	35.7
Colorado	2,260	200.0	723	62.8	350	22.4	407	23.2	484	25.1	393	20.3
Idaho	175	33.4	275	54.2	41	6.6	16	2.4	9	1.3	7	1.0
Montana	173	31.1	64	13.0	183	28.9	167	24.8	133	19.1	92	13.2
Utah	575	104.2	221	34.7	164	20.3	113	12.4	113	11.4	100	10.2
Wyoming	176	71.5	103	40.2	36	11.7	14	4.2	60	17.8	84	25.1
Region VIII	3,359	111.7	1,386	45.5	774	19.7	717	16.5	799	17.2	676	14.6
Alaska	98	132.4	18	22.5	11	6.8	28	13.9	21	9.6	17	7.7
Arizona	607	119.5	400	62.4	1,613	155.9	518	37.8	276	17.7	247	15.6
California	12,796	184.6	10,616	109.3	6,700	51.2	4,877	30.3	7,276	41.0	7,580	41.4
Hawaii	311	78.1	518	107.9	82	15.6	50	8.4	71	11.1	81	12.5
Nevada	236	210.7	268	187.4	89	37.2	97	33.4	234	58.5	177	41.0
Oregon	741	67.4	576	41.3	504	29.4	431	24.0	274	14.7	265	14.0
Washington	1,522	88.2	701	31.2	378	14.6	320	11.3	223	7.6	157	5.4
Region IX	15,902	153.2	12,561	88.8	9,284	49.7	6,321	27.3	8,375	33.0	8,524	32.8
United States	202,984	153.9	121,980	86.5	96,856	58.1	78,264	42.9	67,636	35.7	66,149	34.3
Puerto Rico	---	---	1,590	74.8	1,003	44.5	223	9.5	243	9.5	517	19.7
Virgin Islands	---	---	18	66.7	106	441.7	111	346.9	237	677.1	281	802.9
Canal Zone	---	---	150	312.5	77	197.4	8	22.9	24	68.6	38	108.6
U.S. & Terr.	203,393	153.7	124,274	86.5	98,135	57.8	78,606	42.5	68,140	35.5	66,985	34.2

Note: Alaska and Hawaii included in U.S. & Territories total for fiscal years 1941, 1947, and 1957 and in DHEW Region IX and United States totals beginning with the fiscal year 1962.

Table A.I.8 Civilian cases and rates per 100,000 population for congenital syphilis reported to the Public Health Service by state and territorial health departments; selected fiscal years from 1941 to 1966 (known military cases excluded)

States by DHEW Regions	1941 Cases	1941 Rate	1947 Cases	1947 Rate	1957 Cases	1957 Rate	1962 Cases	1962 Rate	1965 Cases	1965 Rate	1966 Cases	1966 Rate
Connecticut	153	8.9	69	3.7	40	1.8	24	0.9	2	0.1	14	0.5
Maine	68	8.0	33	4.0	-	-	5	0.5	28	2.9	30	3.1
Massachusetts	303	7.0	211	4.8	137	2.9	265	5.1	175	3.3	139	2.6
New Hampshire	35	7.1	26	5.3	8	1.4	3	0.5	3	0.5	10	1.5
Rhode Island	70	9.9	43	5.8	14	1.8	7	0.8	2	0.2	1	0.1
Vermont	14	3.9	20	5.9	4	1.1	-	-	2	0.5	2	0.5
Region I	643	7.6	402	4.6	203	2.1	304	2.9	212	1.9	196	1.8
Delaware	28	10.5	22	7.4	41	10.4	41	9.1	43	8.9	34	6.8
New Jersey	598	14.4	226	5.2	182	3.4	195	3.1	188	2.8	129	1.9
New York	1,671	12.4	819	6.1	421	2.6	294	1.8	281	1.6	309	1.7
Pennsylvania	860	8.7	628	6.4	98	0.9	319	2.8	220	1.9	141	1.2
Region II	3,157	11.4	1,695	6.1	742	2.3	849	2.4	732	2.0	613	1.7
District of Columbia	—	—	125	14.0	37	4.4	38	5.1	72	9.1	40	5.1
Kentucky	199	7.0	183	6.8	87	2.9	53	1.7	76	2.4	88	2.8
Maryland	212	11.6	173	7.8	55	2.0	77	2.5	92	2.7	72	2.1
North Carolina	1,037	29.1	392	10.9	280	6.5	156	3.4	52	1.1	93	1.9
Virginia	639	23.8	343	11.2	169	4.8	164	4.2	119	2.8	101	2.4
West Virginia	210	11.0	310	16.9	90	4.5	32	1.7	42	2.3	57	3.1
Region III	2,297	17.0	1,526	10.7	718	4.4	520	3.0	453	2.5	451	2.5
Alabama	653	23.1	488	16.9	82	2.6	8	0.2	16	0.5	19	0.6
Florida	547	28.6	444	18.7	306	8.3	167	3.2	167	3.0	194	3.4
Georgia	405	13.0	446	13.9	159	4.4	83	2.1	40	1.0	53	1.2
Mississippi	1,837	84.5	929	46.5	94	4.5	31	1.4	25	1.1	16	0.7
South Carolina	367	19.4	214	11.5	517	22.5	107	4.5	74	3.0	92	3.7
Tennessee	794	27.1	299	9.8	113	3.3	54	1.5	46	1.2	35	0.9
Region IV	4,603	31.0	2,820	18.3	1,271	7.0	450	2.2	368	1.7	409	1.9
Illinois	860	10.9	572	7.1	299	3.2	312	3.1	174	1.7	245	2.3
Indiana	352	10.3	251	6.9	113	2.6	90	1.9	64	1.3	45	0.9
Michigan	460	8.7	507	8.7	193	2.6	145	1.8	183	2.3	210	2.6
Ohio	889	12.8	578	7.7	318	3.5	139	1.4	212	2.1	225	2.2
Wisconsin	36	1.1	70	2.2	60	1.6	32	0.8	39	1.0	73	1.8
Region V	2,5__	_._	1,9__	7.6	9__	_._	7__	_._	6__	_._	7_8	2._

Iowa	122	4.8	52	2.2	84	3.1	53	1.9	42	1.5	39	1.4
Kansas	131	7.3	134	7.8	74	3.6	54	2.5	35	1.6	30	1.4
Minnesota	96	3.4	54	2.0	4	0.1	7	0.2	8	0.2	5	0.1
Missouri	375	9.9	326	8.8	172	4.1	144	3.3	168	3.8	130	2.9
Nebraska	40	3.1	72	5.9	31	2.2	26	1.8	22	1.5	27	1.9
North Dakota	33	5.2	8	1.5	1	0.2	-	-	-	-	1	0.2
South Dakota	33	5.2	18	3.3	13	1.9	7	1.0	12	1.7	2	0.3
Region VI	830	6.2	664	5.2	379	2.5	291	1.9	287	1.8	234	1.5
Arkansas	251	12.9	492	28.0	182	10.2	109	6.1	51	2.7	56	2.9
Louisiana	19	0.8	607	24.2	207	7.0	171	5.2	108	3.1	110	3.1
New Mexico	107	20.0	89	16.3	26	3.3	65	6.8	17	1.7	41	4.1
Oklahoma	281	12.2	363	17.1	93	4.2	89	3.8	40	1.6	51	2.1
Texas	1,227	19.2	568	8.1	185	2.1	118	1.2	121	1.2	104	1.0
Region VII	1,885	13.9	2,119	15.2	693	4.2	552	3.1	337	1.8	362	1.9
Colorado	280	24.8	76	6.6	22	1.4	28	1.6	27	1.4	11	0.6
Idaho	20	3.8	30	5.9	7	1.1	-	-	-	-	-	-
Montana	10	1.8	17	3.4	17	2.7	14	2.1	6	0.9	3	0.4
Utah	49	8.9	16	2.5	24	3.0	15	1.6	6	0.6	4	0.4
Wyoming	11	4.5	9	3.5	1	0.3	1	0.3	4	1.2	6	1.8
Region VIII	370	12.3	148	4.9	71	1.8	58	1.3	43	0.9	24	0.5
Alaska	5	6.8	1	1.3	-	-	2	1.0	-	-	1	0.5
Arizona	136	26.8	55	8.6	39	3.8	18	1.3	8	0.5	7	0.4
California	910	13.1	733	7.5	304	2.3	286	1.8	369	2.1	349	1.9
Hawaii	65	16.3	67	14.0	18	3.4	4	0.7	7	1.1	3	0.5
Nevada	30	26.8	22	15.4	6	2.5	5	1.7	2	0.5	3	0.7
Oregon	55	5.0	56	4.0	25	1.5	21	1.2	13	0.7	9	0.5
Washington	87	5.0	53	2.4	18	0.7	7	0.2	2	0.1	5	0.2
Region IX	1,218	11.7	919	6.5	392	2.1	343	1.5	401	1.6	377	1.4
United States	17,600	13.3	12,271	8.7	5,452	3.3	4,085	2.2	3,505	1.9	3,464	1.8
Puerto Rico	-	-	1,765	83.1	125	5.5	17	0.7	11	0.4	38	1.4
Virgin Islands	-	-	4	14.8	2	8.3	2	6.3	-	-	-	-
Canal Zone	-	-	7	14.6	-	-	-	-	-	-	-	-
U.S. & Terr.	17,670	13.4	14,115	9.8	5,597	3.3	4,104	2.2	3,516	1.8	3,502	1.8

Note: Alaska and Hawaii included in U.S. & Territories total for fiscal years 1941, 1947, and 1957 and in DHEW Region IX and United States totals beginning with fiscal year 1962.

Table A.I.9 Civilian cases and rates per 100,000 population for gonorrhea reported to the Public Health Service by state and territorial health departments: selected fiscal years from 1941 to 1966 (known military cases excluded)

States by DHEW Regions	1941 Cases	1941 Rate	1947 Cases	1947 Rate	1957 Cases	1957 Rate	1962 Cases	1962 Rate	1965 Cases	1965 Rate	1966 Cases	1966 Rate
Connecticut	1,273	74.4	1,362	72.1	1,376	61.9	1,777	68.3	2,421	88.0	2,762	97.9
Maine	457	54.0	752	89.4	81	9.1	202	20.7	296	30.5	402	41.2
Massachusetts	3,744	86.5	4,014	90.7	1,529	32.1	2,497	48.2	4,246	80.2	4,401	82.9
New Hampshire	142	28.8	377	77.3	43	7.8	112	18.3	173	26.7	296	44.7
Rhode Island	503	70.8	838	113.2	187	23.5	190	22.5	293	33.0	359	40.1
Vermont	228	63.7	490	143.7	55	15.0	107	27.1	189	46.3	208	52.4
Region I	6,347	75.1	7,833	89.8	3,271	34.1	4,885	46.0	7,618	69.5	8,428	76.2
Delaware	460	172.3	350	117.4	411	104.3	778	172.9	1,055	218.9	1,100	221.3
New Jersey	3,599	86.5	6,612	152.5	4,215	78.7	3,698	59.6	3,882	58.6	4,016	59.6
New York	19,830	147.5	23,081	170.5	13,399	83.0	24,331	145.4	32,946	184.4	37,886	210.2
Pennsylvania	646	6.5	8,323	85.3	4,812	44.0	6,345	56.2	7,918	69.2	8,790	76.4
Region II	24,535	88.2	38,366	137.4	22,837	69.6	35,152	101.3	45,801	125.7	51,795	140.9
District of Columbia	3,407	503.2	12,252	1,376.6	9,732	1,154.5	8,259	1,114.6	10,405	1,310.5	9,941	1,259.9
Kentucky	3,988	140.5	9,935	371.5	3,002	100.6	3,270	107.8	3,410	109.5	3,455	110.0
Maryland	4,197	229.7	6,515	294.8	7,032	256.6	5,868	187.3	6,410	189.5	6,741	194.7
North Carolina	5,360	150.2	13,865	386.1	10,652	245.8	7,716	170.2	9,404	197.5	10,318	214.0
Virginia	3,560	132.7	13,860	451.3	6,751	193.4	6,881	175.4	7,433	176.1	8,060	187.7
West Virginia	3,206	167.9	6,568	358.9	1,065	53.7	1,003	54.2	825	45.9	934	51.6
Region III	23,718	175.7	62,995	441.6	38,234	233.5	32,997	191.7	37,887	209.7	39,449	215.4
Alabama	5,222	184.4	9,027	313.1	3,591	115.5	3,799	115.8	3,647	107.8	4,056	118.0
Florida	2,236	116.9	19,071	805.0	9,997	271.9	9,082	176.7	10,239	182.6	10,619	185.9
Georgia	1,435	46.2	17,151	534.3	12,851	353.5	9,910	252.9	10,969	261.4	12,149	285.0
Mississippi	28,777	1,323.7	33,800	1,692.5	7,497	356.3	5,049	230.5	4,757	207.7	4,401	191.3
South Carolina	1,292	68.4	10,514	562.8	6,235	270.7	9,092	385.9	8,140	326.9	7,121	286.2
Tennessee	4,116	141.7	26,715	875.0	12,915	374.6	8,968	249.3	9,353	248.1	9,962	261.1
Region IV	43,116	290.4	116,278	756.0	53,086	290.5	45,900	224.1	47,105	216.7	48,308	219.4
Illinois	18,483	234.4	34,545	428.3	20,023	213.6	25,757	256.7	26,746	256.1	31,153	294.0
Indiana	1,952	57.0	2,007	55.2	2,040	46.3	3,038	64.6	3,903	81.0	4,540	93.1
Michigan	7,930	150.1	11,327	193.6	8,862	118.1	10,497	132.3	12,896	159.7	14,765	180.1
Ohio	5,921	85.6	9,720	130.2	7,044	77.6	9,939	100.8	13,015	129.0	14,527	142.1
Wisconsin	1,046	33.3	1,401	44.7	832	22.1	1,248	31.1	1,758	42.9	2,362	57.1
Region V	35,332	132.6	59,000	209.6	38,801	113.7	50,479	138.1	58,318	155.4	67,347	177.1

167

Iowa	60.8	1,535	66.4	1,581	23.1	621	47.8	1,327	80.7	2,224	104.2	2,873
Kansas	69.7	1,243	154.3	2,661	78.4	1,615	108.2	2,336	121.1	2,650	127.5	2,798
Minnesota	64.7	1,803	67.4	1,826	22.7	735	53.6	1,858	62.1	2,182	61.6	2,187
Missouri	96.6	3,653	196.1	7,261	123.4	5,214	179.2	7,797	215.9	9,443	192.9	8,622
Nebraska	68.0	890	96.2	1,174	47.8	670	53.3	753	67.4	984	74.0	1,080
North Dakota	66.1	421	73.2	396	28.7	188	93.5	591	92.1	584	69.1	442
South Dakota	39.9	254	99.6	550	64.3	443	144.3	990	130.9	927	94.7	659
Region VI	72.8	9,799	120.4	15,449	63.4	9,486	101.1	15,652	121.5	18,994	118.4	18,661
Arkansas	95.2	1,850	408.2	7,164	260.4	4,668	426.0	7,616	332.7	6,381	311.0	6,064
Louisiana	72.8	1,721	526.9	13,242	191.4	5,668	172.7	5,703	145.2	4,986	157.4	5,509
New Mexico	97.0	518	257.7	1,407	108.9	861	131.8	1,268	168.8	1,666	155.6	1,567
Oklahoma	187.2	4,317	425.6	9,040	183.2	4,040	206.6	4,812	137.8	3,352	140.8	3,446
Texas	173.8	11,119	342.3	23,957	158.8	13,881	237.4	22,825	267.2	27,325	275.0	28,560
Region VII	144.2	19,525	393.3	54,810	176.6	29,118	234.6	42,224	230.1	43,710	234.0	45,146
Colorado	116.2	1,313	193.3	2,225	49.7	775	99.8	1,752	106.0	2,041	113.6	2,195
Idaho	23.5	123	130.2	660	40.7	253	70.2	476	117.8	808	152.9	1,049
Montana	41.7	232	64.4	318	36.5	231	56.1	378	60.0	417	68.0	473
Utah	85.1	470	66.7	425	28.3	229	38.5	351	47.7	471	43.4	427
Wyoming	161.8	398	79.3	203	20.4	63	20.6	69	44.7	151	47.8	160
Region VIII	84.3	2,536	125.8	3,831	39.5	1,551	69.5	3,026	83.9	3,888	92.9	4,304
Alaska	477.0	353	996.3	797	146.0	149	277.6	558	287.6	627	470.6	1,040
Arizona	364.2	1,850	246.6	1,581	200.6	2,076	184.8	2,533	195.2	3,047	199.1	3,158
California	300.4	20,825	349.9	33,998	123.0	16,106	142.3	22,912	204.9	36,376	220.0	40,243
Hawaii	272.6	1,085	140.4	674	28.3	235	30.0	179	50.4	323	62.0	402
Nevada	131.9	149	337.8	483	110.0	263	156.6	454	200.0	800	159.0	687
Oregon	112.4	1,236	146.5	2,042	30.1	516	64.0	1,148	122.8	2,290	133.7	2,532
Washington	260.9	4,500	176.7	3,973	43.6	1,131	83.4	2,369	115.1	3,371	117.8	3,449
Region IX	275.2	28,560	297.5	42,077	107.6	20,064	130.0	30,153	184.6	46,834	198.1	51,511
United States	146.7	193,468	284.2	400,639	129.8	216,448	142.8	260,468	163.3	310,155	173.6	334,949
Puerto Rico	---	---	303.6	6,452	146.7	3,310	110.2	2,577	107.6	2,760	105.9	2,781
Virgin Islands	---	---	811.1	219	429.2	103	496.9	159	714.3	250	1,074.3	376
Canal Zone	---	---	2,072.9	995	874.4	341	922.9	323	937.1	328	634.3	222
U.S. & Terr.	147.5	194,906	285.1	409,776	129.9	220,614	142.6	263,527	163.3	313,493	172.9	338,328

Note: Alaska and Hawaii included in U.S. & Territories total for fiscal years 1941, 1947, and 1957 and in DHEW Region IX and United States totals beginning with fiscal year 1962.

Table A.I.10 Civilian cases and rates per 100,000 population for all stages of syphilis in cities with over 200,000 population: selected fiscal years from 1957 to 1966 (known military cases excluded)

Cities by DHEW Regions	1957 Cases	1957 Rate	1962 Cases	1962 Rate	1965 Cases	1965 Rate	1966 Cases	1966 Rate
Boston	887	110.7	1,487	215.8	1,117	169.2	900	138.1
Providence	249	100.0	126	62.1	217	109.0	183	92.0
Buffalo[a]	402	44.7	314	29.3	305	26.9	487	42.5
Jersey City	235	78.6	548	200.0	329	121.9	270	101.1
Newark	1,681	382.9	1,482	368.7	1,494	380.1	1,043	267.5
New York City	16,619	210.6	20,068	258.4	17,281	223.2	16,123	205.9
Philadelphia	2,040	98.5	5,186	260.0	2,148	108.2	2,024	99.2
Pittsburgh[a]	639	94.4	1,696	103.4	923	55.4	726	43.7
Rochester[a]	161	48.5	222	37.6	103	16.5	115	18.2
Syracuse	120	54.3	46	21.4	116	54.0	104	48.4
Baltimore	1,346	141.7	1,601	171.6	1,647	176.6	1,749	189.0
Charlotte	--	--	278	134.3	127	56.7	160	69.3
Louisville[a]	553	149.9	484	78.4	501	75.3	520	78.1
Norfolk	459	214.5	497	158.8	237	73.4	294	91.0
Richmond	547	237.8	475	217.9	322	145.6	208	92.4
Washington, D. C.	1,957	232.2	1,927	260.1	1,728	217.7	1,473	186.7
Atlanta[a]	713	150.4	745	130.5	499	85.2	643	107.7
Birmingham	888	272.4	603	176.8	594	172.6	477	137.8
Jacksonville[b]	658	321.0	806	399.0	659	130.4	795	153.5
Memphis[a]	587	121.8	667	104.5	818	119.2	576	81.4
Miami[a]	942	378.3	1,056	354.4	851	76.9	1,294	115.6
Mobile[a]	--	--	247	76.9	326	94.2	358	101.4
Tampa[b]	--	--	479	168.1	417	94.2	399	87.5
Akron	212	77.1	131	45.2	205	69.0	147	50.1
Chicago	3,816	105.4	6,391	181.1	5,198	147.1	6,006	169.4
Cincinnati	892	177.0	476	95.2	574	114.8	373	74.6
Cleveland	887	96.9	470	54.0	916	105.3	861	99.6
Columbus	541	143.9	295	61.7	381	74.0	408	76.6
Dayton	275	112.7	218	82.9	247	93.2	173	65.0

Detroit	2,812	152.0	1,432	86.8	3,260	201.9	3,777	235.8
Indianapolis	638	149.4	612	125.4	512	99.7	461	89.4
Milwaukee	500	78.5	248	33.2	473	61.9	788	101.7
Toledo	450	148.0	230	72.3	205	64.5	197	53.1
Des Moines	---	---	198	93.8	170	79.2	229	105.6
Kansas City	1,007	220.4	1,268	266.4	1,010	189.8	935	173.2
Minneapolis[a]	72	13.8	126	26.3	129	14.4	84	9.4
Omaha	168	66.9	155	50.0	144	44.1	131	38.3
St. Louis	2,863	334.1	1,710	230.8	1,723	239.3	1,194	167.9
St. Paul	22	7.1	36	11.5	26	8.3	32	10.1
Wichita[a]	---	---	138	39.1	95	27.1	108	31.4
Albuquerque[a]	---	---	224	82.7	117	39.7	278	116.8
Dallas[a]	468	107.8	387	55.4	398	35.6	529	45.3
El Paso[a]	76	---	224	68.9	275	76.8	276	77.8
Fort Worth[a]	---	27.2	231	64.2	207	34.2	168	28.2
Houston[a]	1,260	211.4	2,005	157.3	2,239	158.2	2,297	158.1
New Orleans	2,313	405.8	1,984	313.9	878	134.7	1,113	167.7
Oklahoma City[a]	215	88.1	307	93.0	345	69.8	247	47.7
San Antonio[a]	58	14.2	106	17.6	560	72.9	534	69.6
Tulsa[a]	---	---	148	41.9	154	40.6	220	57.1
Denver[a]	304	73.1	308	61.6	294	56.1	295	55.9
Honolulu	67	27.2	64	21.6	59	17.6	76	22.3
Long Beach[b]	196	78.1	215	61.4	297	82.3		---
Los Angeles[b]	1,674	85.0	2,643	105.4	5,760	215.1	6,395	93.7
Oakland[a]	137	35.6	299	38.2	477	54.8	578	63.8
Phoenix[a]	---	---	339	49.7	211	26.1	195	22.5
Portland	203	54.3	222	59.7	152	40.2	165	43.3
San Diego[a]	139	25.0	233	21.9	172	14.5	183	15.3
San Francisco	547	70.6	1,035	140.2	953	127.9	927	124.9
San Jose	---	---	88	41.5	140	47.2	135	42.2
Seattle[a]	175	23.9	190	20.0	181	17.7	121	12.0
Tucson[a]	---	---	151	55.5	97	31.0	112	34.4
San Juan[a]	388	172.4	226	32.5	720	98.3	929	124.2

a County data.
b Jacksonville, Miami, Tampa: county data beginning in 1965. Los Angeles: county data in 1966.

Table A.I.11   Civilian cases and rates per 100,000 population for primary and secondary syphilis reported to the Public Health Service by cities with over 200,000 population: selected fiscal years from 1957 to 1966 (known military cases excluded)

Cities by DHEW Regions	1957 Cases	1957 Rate	1962 Cases	1962 Rate	1965 Cases	1965 Rate	1966 Cases	1966 Rate
Boston	124	15.5	218	31.6	158	23.9	217	33.3
Providence	2	0.8	10	4.9	9	4.5	25	12.6
Buffalo[a]	23	2.6	75	7.0	30	2.6	38	3.3
Jersey City	12	4.0	36	13.1	83	30.7	80	30.0
Newark	37	8.4	379	94.3	324	82.4	279	71.5
New York City	576	7.3	3,307	42.6	2,931	37.9	2,819	36.0
Philadelphia	85	4.1	735	36.8	274	13.8	361	17.7
Pittsburgh[a]	19	2.8	63	3.8	19	1.1	58	3.5
Rochester[a]	8	2.4	77	13.0	27	4.3	26	4.1
Syracuse	22	10.0	11	5.1	18	8.4	26	12.1
Baltimore	196	20.6	419	44.9	345	37.0	412	44.5
Charlotte	—	—	90	43.5	77	34.4	80	34.6
Louisville[a]	7	1.9	103	16.7	80	12.0	42	6.3
Norfolk	25	11.7	76	24.3	31	9.6	19	5.9
Richmond	29	12.6	67	30.7	39	17.6	28	12.4
Washington, D. C.	106	12.6	702	94.7	551	69.4	468	59.3
Atlanta[a]	82	17.3	210	36.8	175	29.9	225	37.7
Birmingham	25	7.7	90	26.4	168	48.8	196	56.6
Jacksonville[b]	20	9.8	194	96.0	137	27.1	159	30.7
Memphis[a]	36	7.5	25	3.9	144	21.0	82	11.6
Miami[b]	41	16.5	286	96.0	229	20.7	357	31.9
Mobile[a]	—	—	108	33.6	193	55.8	210	59.5
Tampa[b]	—	—	141	49.5	139	31.4	88	19.3
Akron	15	5.5	25	8.6	58	19.5	17	5.8
Chicago	398	11.0	858	24.3	1,158	32.8	1,082	30.5
Cincinnati	21	4.2	18	3.6	80	16.0	95	19.0
Cleveland	31	3.4	95	10.9	251	28.9	274	31.7
Columbus	2	0.5	21	4.4	38	7.4	43	8.1
Dayton	10	4.1	17	6.5	16	6.0	10	3.8
Detroit	41	2.2	178	10.8	551	34.1	867	54.1

Indianapolis	14	3.3	50	10.2	39	7.6	24	4.7
Milwaukee	16	2.5	17	2.3	51	6.7	60	7.7
Toledo	3	1.0	14	4.4	52	16.4	35	9.4
Des Moines	—	—	4	1.9	7	3.3	31	14.3
Kansas City	26	5.7	47	9.9	40	7.5	40	7.4
Minneapolis[a]	12	2.3	37	7.7	62	6.9	23	2.6
Omaha	—	—	5	1.6	5	1.5	11	3.2
St. Louis	27	3.2	102	13.8	192	26.7	126	17.7
St. Paul	1	0.3	16	5.1	16	5.1	6	1.9
Wichita[a]	—	—	9	2.5	3	0.9	24	7.0
Albuquerque[a]	—	—	19	7.0	48	16.3	24	10.1
Dallas[a]	76	17.5	146	20.9	125	11.2	181	15.5
El Paso[a]	16	5.7	45	13.8	92	25.7	71	20.0
Fort Worth[a]	172	28.5	95	26.4	89	14.7	90	15.1
Houston[a]	19	3.3	579	45.4	310	21.9	368	25.3
New Orleans	10	4.1	642	101.6	207	31.7	102	15.4
Oklahoma City[a]	13	3.2	23	7.0	68	13.8	40	7.7
San Antonio[a]	—	—	21	3.5	56	7.3	60	7.8
Tulsa[a]	—	—	16	4.5	32	8.4	38	9.9
Denver[a]	17	4.1	40	8.0	21	4.0	14	2.7
Honolulu	1	0.4	11	3.7	18	5.4	30	8.8
Long Beach	5	2.0	31	8.9	34	9.4	—	—
Los Angeles[b]	113	5.7	646	25.8	917	34.2	839	12.3
Oakland[a]	8	2.1	60	7.7	81	9.3	79	8.7
Phoenix[a]	—	—	58	8.5	83	10.3	75	8.7
Portland	10	2.7	26	7.0	20	5.3	19	5.0
San Diego[a]	10	1.8	49	4.6	43	3.6	61	5.1
San Francisco	124	16.0	246	33.3	265	35.6	190	25.6
San Jose	—	—	16	7.5	17	5.7	17	5.3
Seattle[a]	13	1.8	31	3.3	47	4.6	36	5.3
Tucson	—	—	31	11.4	44	14.1	39	12.0
San Juan[a]	18	8.0	62	8.9	403	55.0	422	56.4

a County data.
b Jacksonville, Miami, Tampa: county data beginning in 1965. Los Angeles: county data in 1966.

Table A.I.12 Civilian cases and rates per 100,000 population for early latent syphilis reported to the Public Health Service by cities with over 200,000 population: selected fiscal years from 1957 to 1966 (known military cases excluded)

Cities by DHEW Regions	1957 Cases	1957 Rate	1962 Cases	1962 Rate	1965 Cases	1965 Rate	1966 Cases	1966 Rate
Boston	136	17.0	141	20.4	147	22.3	148	22.7
Providence	13	5.2	14	6.9	8	4.0	19	9.5
Buffalo[a]	14	1.6	32	3.0	17	1.5	18	1.6
Jersey City	33	11.0	56	20.4	75	27.8	77	28.8
Newark	144	32.8	231	57.5	359	91.3	180	46.2
New York City	1,672	21.2	3,886	50.0	4,162	53.8	4,048	51.7
Philadelphia[a]	332	16.0	585	29.3	176	8.9	131	6.4
Pittsburgh[a]	85	12.6	65	4.0	19	1.1	11	0.7
Rochester[a]	1	0.3	28	4.7	12	1.9	8	1.3
Syracuse	9	4.1	6	2.8	8	3.7	15	7.0
Baltimore	64	6.7	309	33.1	304	32.6	375	40.5
Charlotte			50	24.2	15	6.7	26	11.3
Louisville[a]	11	3.0	20	3.2	20	3.0	38	5.7
Norfolk	75	35.1	67	21.4	29	9.0	36	11.1
Richmond	68	29.6	19	8.7	17	7.7	14	6.2
Washington, D. C.	298	35.4	329	44.4	363	45.7	327	41.4
Atlanta[a]	194	40.9	207	36.3	123	21.0	156	26.1
Birmingham	231	70.9	159	46.6	111	32.3	53	15.3
Jacksonville[b]	189	92.2	245	121.3	63	12.5	76	14.7
Memphis[a]	88	18.3	34	5.3	109	15.9	76	10.7
Miami[b]	266	106.8	428	143.6	191	17.3	241	21.5
Mobile[a]			105	32.7	100	28.9	89	25.2
Tampa[b]			74	26.0	41	9.3	30	6.6
Akron	20	7.3	12	4.1	13	4.4	14	4.8
Chicago	806	22.3	1,400	39.7	999	28.3	1,117	31.5
Cincinnati	196	38.9	67	13.4	39	7.8	35	7.0
Cleveland	222	24.3	91	10.5	209	24.0	237	27.4
Columbus	25	6.7	15	3.1	29	5.6	39	7.3
Dayton	57	23.4	37	14.1	33	12.5	17	6.4
Detroit	491	26.5	87	5.3	208	12.9	357	22.3
Indianapolis	61	14.3	63	12.9	45	8.3	39	7.6
Milwaukee	76	11.9	28	3.7	73	9.5	85	11.0
Toledo	26	8.6	15	4.7	16	5.0	16	4.3

Des Moines			2	0.9	1	0.5	3	1.4
Kansas City	83	18.2	86	18.1	42	7.9	50	9.3
Minneapolis[a]	10	1.9	18	3.3	14	1.6	20	2.2
Omaha	7	2.3	14	4.5	9	2.8	13	3.8
St. Louis	271	31.6	226	30.5	150	20.8	96	13.5
St. Paul	3	1.0	6	1.9	1	0.3	7	2.2
Wichita[a]			11	3.1	5	1.4	14	4.1
Albuquerque[a]	67	15.4	9	3.3	9	3.1	6	2.5
Dallas[a]			80	11.5	95	8.5	95	8.1
El Paso[a]	27	9.7	95	29.2	60	16.8	56	15.8
Fort Worth[a]	265	44.5	67	18.6	69	11.4	59	9.9
Houston[a]	153	26.8	631	49.5	517	36.5	439	30.2
New Orleans	24	9.8	209	33.1	95	14.6	112	16.9
Oklahoma City[a]	13	3.2	36	10.9	20	4.0	27	5.2
San Antonio[a]			30	5.0	91	11.8	137	17.9
Tulsa[a]			10	2.8	23	6.1	29	7.5
Denver[a]	60	14.4	24	4.8	30	5.7	21	4.0
Honolulu	5	2.0	9	3.0	3	0.9	9	2.6
Long Beach	17	6.8	26	7.4	35	9.7		
Los Angeles[b]	318	16.1	498	19.9	1,041	34.2	1,167	17.1
Oakland[a]	21	5.5	85	10.9	64	7.3	116	12.8
Phoenix[a]	35	9.4	63	9.2	30	3.7	26	3.0
Portland	34	6.1	15	4.0	6	1.6	17	4.5
San Diego[a]	126	16.3	48	4.5	44	3.7	20	1.7
San Francisco			282	38.2	338	45.4	317	42.7
San Jose	20	2.7	14	6.6	15	5.1	13	4.1
Seattle[a]			31	3.3	33	3.2	21	2.1
Tucson[a]			55	20.2	22	7.0	26	8.0
San Juan[a]	45	20.0	89	12.8	184	25.1	280	37.4

[a] County data.
[b] Jacksonville, Miami, Tampa: county data beginning in 1965. Los Angeles: county data in 1966.

Table A.I.13   Civilian cases and rates per 100,000 population for late and late latent syphilis reported to the Public Health Service by cities with over 200,000 population: selected fiscal years from 1957 to 1966 (known military cases excluded)

Cities by DHEW Regions	1957 Cases	1957 Rate	1962 Cases	1962 Rate	1965 Cases	1965 Rate	1966 Cases	1966 Rate
Boston	578	72.2	1,016	147.2	738	111.8	482	74.0
Providence	180	72.3	67	33.0	101	50.8	77	38.7
Buffalo[a]	348	38.7	202	18.8	255	22.5	411	35.9
Jersey City	176	58.9	449	163.9	160	59.3	106	39.7
Newark	1,437	327.3	822	204.5	747	190.1	544	139.5
New York City	14,061	178.2	12,653	162.9	9,969	128.8	9,030	115.3
Philadelphia	1,568	75.7	3,744	187.7	1,641	82.6	1,487	72.9
Pittsburgh[a]	511	75.5	1,527	93.1	860	51.7	650	39.1
Rochester[a]	141	42.5	109	18.4	61	9.8	76	12.0
Syracuse[a]	86	38.9	28	13.0	81	37.7	57	26.5
Baltimore	940	99.0	745	79.8	943	101.1	895	96.8
Charlotte	--	--	130	62.8	34	15.2	46	19.9
Louisville[a]	504	136.6	306	49.6	304	45.7	361	54.2
Norfolk	341	159.4	322	102.9	159	49.2	232	71.8
Richmond	419	182.2	355	162.8	225	101.8	149	66.2
Washington, D. C.	1,515	179.7	857	115.7	709	89.3	638	80.9
Atlanta[a]	326	68.8	310	54.3	198	33.8	248	41.5
Birmingham	572	175.5	346	101.5	307	89.2	220	63.6
Jacksonville[b]	432	210.7	346	171.3	440	87.0	533	102.9
Memphis[a]	447	92.7	593	92.9	550	80.1	411	58.1
Miami[b]	606	243.4	317	106.4	404	36.5	673	60.1
Mobile[a]	--	--	32	10.0	32	9.2	57	16.1
Tampa[b]	--	--	247	86.7	214	48.3	258	56.6
Akron	155	56.4	88	30.3	131	44.1	106	36.1
Chicago	2,395	66.1	3,876	109.8	2,893	81.8	3,607	101.8
Cincinnati	646	128.2	373	74.6	435	87.0	233	46.6
Cleveland	616	67.3	270	31.0	442	50.8	331	38.3
Columbus	173	125.8	236	49.4	292	56.7	304	57.1

	(1)	(2)	(3)	(4)	(5)	(6)	(7)	(8)
Dayton	194	79.5	161	61.2	179	67.5	127	47.7
Detroit	1,616	87.4	936	56.7	2,294	142.1	2,323	145.0
Indianapolis	519	121.6	469	96.1	408	79.4	379	73.4
Milwaukee	301	47.3	162	21.7	324	42.4	560	72.3
Toledo	398	130.9	195	61.3	130	40.9	128	34.5
Des Moines	—	—	182	86.3	152	70.7	186	85.7
Kansas City	867	189.7	1,083	227.5	877	164.8	801	148.3
Minneapolis[a]	50	9.6	66	13.7	49	5.5	39	4.4
Omaha	150	59.8	124	40.0	121	37.0	96	28.1
St. Louis	2,477	289.0	1,339	180.7	1,307	181.5	910	128.0
St. Paul	17	5.5	12	3.8	9	2.9	18	5.7
Wichita[a]	—	—	108	30.6	81	23.1	65	18.8
Albuquerque[a]	325	74.9	183	67.5	57	19.3	234	98.3
Dallas[a]	—	—	158	22.6	178	15.9	252	21.6
El Paso[a]	32	11.5	76	23.4	114	31.8	138	38.9
Fort Worth[a]	755	126.7	69	19.2	46	7.6	19	3.2
Houston[a]	1,937	339.8	733	57.5	1,348	95.3	1,445	99.5
New Orleans	167	68.4	1,075	170.1	547	83.9	856	128.9
Oklahoma City[a]	24	5.9	235	71.2	247	50.0	166	32.1
San Antonio[a]	—	—	48	8.0	404	52.6	326	42.5
Tulsa[a]	—	—	109	30.9	90	23.7	140	36.4
Denver[a]	219	52.6	233	46.6	231	44.1	252	47.7
Honolulu	48	19.5	39	13.2	35	10.4	36	10.6
Long Beach	159	63.4	154	44.0	226	62.6	—	—
Los Angeles[b]	1,122	57.0	1,404	56.0	3,580	133.7	4,168	61.1
Oakland[a]	92	23.9	147	18.8	321	36.9	369	40.8
Phoenix[a]	—	—	207	30.4	94	11.6	92	10.6
Portland	148	39.6	170	45.7	118	31.2	122	32.0
San Diego[a]	90	16.2	134	12.6	82	6.9	83	6.9
San Francisco	274	35.4	486	65.9	337	45.2	406	54.7
San Jose	—	—	47	22.2	100	33.7	94	29.4
Seattle[a]	138	18.8	125	13.2	100	9.8	64	6.3
Tucson[a]	—	—	62	22.8	31	9.9	45	13.8
San Juan[a]	304	135.1	73	10.5	131	17.9	217	29.0

[a] County data.
[b] Jacksonville, Miami, Tampa: county data beginning in 1965. Los Angeles: county data in 1966.

Table A.I.14 Civilian cases and rates per 100,000 population for congenital syphilis reported to the Public Health Service by cities with over 200,000 population: selected fiscal years from 1957 to 1966 (known military cases excluded)

Cities by DHEW Regions	1957		1962		1965		1966	
	Cases	Rate	Cases	Rate	Cases	Rate	Cases	Rate
Boston	44	5.5	114	16.5	74	11.2	53	8.1
Providence	4	1.6	3	1.5	-	-	-	-
Buffalo[a]	17	1.9	5	0.5	3	0.3	20	1.7
Jersey City	14	4.7	7	2.6	11	4.1	7	2.6
Newark	61	13.9	50	12.4	64	16.3	40	10.3
New York City	310	3.9	222	2.9	219	2.8	226	2.9
Philadelphia	55	2.7	122	6.1	57	2.9	45	2.2
Pittsburgh[a]	24	3.6	41	2.5	25	1.5	7	0.4
Rochester[a]	11	3.3	8	1.4	3	0.5	5	0.8
Syracuse	3	1.4	1	0.5	9	4.2	6	2.8
Baltimore	29	3.1	31	3.3	30	3.2	30	3.2
Charlotte	-	-	8	3.9	1	0.4	8	3.5
Louisville[a]	27	7.3	8	1.3	23	3.5	17	2.6
Norfolk	11	5.1	19	6.1	8	2.5	7	2.2
Richmond	17	7.4	18	8.3	16	7.2	8	3.6
Washington, D. C.	37	4.4	38	5.1	72	9.1	40	5.1
Atlanta[a]	15	3.2	4	0.7	3	0.5	13	2.2
Birmingham	25	7.7	8	2.3	8	2.3	7	2.0
Jacksonville[b]	17	8.3	21	10.4	19	3.8	27	5.2
Memphis[a]	16	3.3	15	2.4	15	2.2	7	1.0
Miami[b]	29	11.7	25	8.4	27	2.4	23	2.1
Mobile[a]	-	-	1	0.3	1	0.3	2	0.6
Tampa[b]	-	-	17	6.0	23	5.2	23	5.0
Akron	22	7.9	6	2.1	3	1.0	10	3.4
Chicago	217	6.0	257	7.3	148	4.2	200	5.6
Cincinnati	29	5.8	18	3.6	20	4.0	20	2.0
Cleveland	13	2.0	14	1.6	14	1.6	19	2.2
Columbus	41	10.9	23	4.8	22	4.3	22	4.1
Dayton	14	5.7	3	1.1	19	7.2	19	7.1
Detroit	109	5.9	52	3.2	90	5.6	107	6.7

Indianapolis	41	9.6	30	6.1	20	3.9	19	3.7
Milwaukee	25	3.9	19	2.5	16	2.1	37	4.8
Toledo	23	7.6	6	1.9	7	2.2	18	4.9
Des Moines	—	—	7	3.3	7	3.3	6	2.8
Kansas City	31	6.8	47	9.9	42	7.9	29	5.4
Minneapolis[a]	—	—	5	1.0	4	0.4	2	0.2
Omaha	9	3.6	12	3.9	9	2.8	11	3.2
St. Louis	88	10.3	36	4.9	57	7.9	57	8.0
St. Paul	1	0.3	1	0.3	0	0.0	1	0.3
Wichita[a]	—	—	9	2.5	6	1.7	3	0.9
Albuquerque[a]	—	—	12	4.4	3	1.0	14	5.9
Dallas[a]	—	—	—	—	—	—	1	0.1
El Paso[a]	1	0.4	8	2.5	9	2.5	11	3.1
Fort Worth[a]	—	—	—	—	3	0.5	—	—
Houston[a]	68	11.4	62	4.9	64	4.5	45	3.1
New Orleans	44	7.7	46	7.3	26	4.0	36	5.4
Oklahoma City[a]	14	5.7	13	3.9	8	1.6	13	2.5
San Antonio[a]	8	2.0	7	1.2	9	1.2	11	1.4
Tulsa[a]	—	—	13	3.7	6	1.6	9	2.3
Denver[a]	8	1.9	11	2.2	12	2.3	8	1.5
Honolulu	13	5.3	4	1.4	3	0.9	1	0.3
Long Beach	12	4.8	4	1.1	2	0.6	—	—
Los Angeles[b]	114	5.8	95	3.8	222	8.3	221	3.2
Oakland[a]	7	1.8	7	0.9	11	1.3	14	1.5
Phoenix[a]	—	—	11	1.6	4	0.5	2	0.2
Portland	9	2.4	4	1.1	6	1.6	5	1.3
San Diego[a]	5	0.9	2	0.2	3	0.3	19	1.6
San Francisco	11	1.4	20	2.7	13	1.7	14	1.9
San Jose	—	—	8	3.8	8	2.7	11	3.4
Seattle[a]	4	0.6	3	0.3	1	0.1	—	—
Tucson[a]	—	—	3	1.1	—	—	2	0.6
San Juan[a]	21	9.3	2	0.3	2	0.3	8	1.1

a County data.
b Jacksonville, Miami, Tampa: county data beginning in 1965. Los Angeles: county data in 1966.

Table A.I.15   Civilian cases and rates per 100,000 population for gonorrhea reported to the Public Health Service by cities with over 200,000 population: selected fiscal years from 1957 to 1966 (known military cases excluded)

Cities by DHEW Regions	1957 Cases	1957 Rate	1962 Cases	1962 Rate	1965 Cases	1965 Rate	1966 Cases	1966 Rate
Boston	957	119.5	1,638	237.4	2,926	443.3	2,812	432.0
Providence	149	59.8	122	60.1	166	83.4	227	114.1
Buffalo[a]	625	69.5	1,250	116.5	1,388	122.4	1,858	162.4
Jersey City	225	75.3	338	123.4	209	77.4	178	66.7
Newark	2,078	473.4	1,524	379.1	2,125	540.7	2,248	576.4
New York City	10,695	135.5	19,209	247.1	26,726	345.3	30,002	383.2
Philadelphia	3,883	187.4	4,974	249.3	5,984	301.2	6,637	325.3
Pittsburgh[a]	609	90.0	720	43.9	898	53.9	1,038	62.4
Rochester[a]	332	100.0	673	113.9	1,032	165.7	1,337	211.2
Syracuse	333	150.7	535	248.8	635	295.3	683	317.7
Baltimore	6,726	708.0	5,503	589.8	5,599	600.1	5,941	642.3
Charlotte	986	267.2	1,384	668.6	1,868	833.9	2,291	991.8
Louisville[a]	2,788	1,302.8	1,779	288.3	1,932	290.5	1,931	289.9
Norfolk	662	287.8	1,300	415.3	1,235	382.4	1,589	492.0
Richmond			1,051	482.1	1,285	581.4	1,483	659.1
Washington, D. C.	9,732	1,154.5	8,259	1,114.6	10,405	1,310.5	9,941	1,259.9
Atlanta[a]	6,840	1,443.0	5,784	1,013.0	7,171	1,223.7	7,848	1,314.6
Birmingham	981	300.9	1,060	310.9	1,264	367.4	1,398	404.0
Jacksonville[b]	1,911	932.2	1,526	755.4	1,102	217.8	1,002	193.4
Memphis[a]	6,487	1,345.9	4,908	769.3	5,035	732.9	5,310	750.0
Miami[b]	1,325	532.1	1,959	657.4	1,870	168.9	2,216	197.9
Mobile[a]	—	—	1,115	347.4	1,138	328.9	1,252	354.7
Tampa[b]	—	—	1,137	398.9	1,690	381.5	1,904	417.5
Akron	510	185.5	724	249.7	1,401	471.7	2,000	680.3
Chicago	17,783	491.1	22,520	638.1	22,755	643.7	26,077	736.0
Cincinnati	1,108	219.8	1,722	344.4	1,633	326.6	1,312	262.4
Cleveland	2,083	227.7	3,081	354.1	4,147	476.7	4,186	484.5
Columbus	718	191.0	1,140	238.5	2,078	403.5	2,320	436.1
Dayton	558	228.7	1,371	521.3	1,052	397.0	1,167	438.7
Detroit	5,655	305.7	6,281	380.7	6,739	417.5	7,202	449.6
Indianapolis	1,295	303.3	1,775	363.7	2,172	422.6	2,362	457.8
Milwaukee	708	111.2	1,009	134.9	1,234	161.3	1,750	225.8
Toledo	291	95.7	370	116.4	459	144.3	543	146.4

	1	2	3	4	5	6	7	8
Des Moines	—	—	491	232.7	522	242.8	626	288.5
Kansas City	629	137.6	2,149	451.5	2,671	502.1	2,806	519.6
Minneapolis[a]	373	71.5	976	203.3	1,097	122.8	1,031	115.5
Omaha	410	163.4	421	135.8	578	176.8	661	193.3
St. Louis	3,800	443.4	4,914	663.2	5,783	803.2	4,560	641.4
St. Paul	139	44.7	349	111.9	430	136.9	429	136.6
Wichita[a]	—	—	709	200.8	791	225.4	838	242.9
Albuquerque[a]	—	—	449	165.7	402	136.3	399	167.6
Dallas[a]	3,203	738.0	4,723	676.6	6,679	595.8	7,591	651.0
El Paso[a]	999	358.1	626	192.6	779	217.6	627	176.6
Fort Worth[a]	2,605	437.1	2,757	765.8	3,883	642.9	4,017	671.7
Houston[a]	2,207	387.2	5,293	415.1	7,196	508.6	7,497	516.3
New Orleans	1,761	721.7	2,078	328.8	1,767	271.0	1,765	265.8
Oklahoma City[a]	452	110.8	1,772	537.0	1,347	272.7	1,415	273.7
San Antonio[a]	—	—	856	142.2	1,109	144.4	1,240	161.7
Tulsa[a]	—	—	298	84.4	362	95.3	346	89.9
Denver[a]	578	138.9	1,429	285.8	1,625	310.1	1,726	326.9
Honolulu	96	39.0	126	42.6	219	65.2	296	86.8
Long Beach	340	135.5	515	147.1	951	263.4	—	—
Los Angeles[b]	6,751	342.7	8,228	328.2	16,057	599.6	16,792	246.1
Oakland[a]	1,345	349.4	1,443	184.3	2,162	248.2	2,464	272.6
Phoenix[a]	242	64.7	1,324	194.1	1,850	229.0	1,785	206.4
Portland	725	130.2	536	144.1	1,038	274.6	1,234	323.9
San Diego[a]	1,709	220.5	811	76.3	1,231	103.1	1,388	115.6
San Francisco	—	—	3,376	457.5	5,242	703.6	6,833	920.9
San Jose	—	—	246	116.0	448	150.8	482	150.6
Seattle[a]	636	86.8	1,432	150.9	2,032	200.0	2,089	206.4
Tucson[a]	—	—	500	183.8	255	81.5	367	112.9
San Juan[a]	1,059	470.7	781	112.1	1,671	228.0	1,779	237.8

[a] County data.
[b] Jacksonville, Miami, Tampe: county data beginning in 1965. Los Angeles: county data in 1966.

Table A.I.16   Reported cases of congenital syphilis by age: United States, fiscal years 1951-66

Fiscal Year	Total			Distribution of known ages				Estimated Less than one years[a]
	All ages	Unknown ages	Known ages	Less than 1 year	1 - 4 years	5 - 9 years	Over 10 years	
1951	12,836	1,528	11,308	701	817	2,003	7,787	796
1952	9,240	1,051	8,189	551	426	1,104	6,108	622
1953	8,021	1,542	6,479	331	265	749	5,134	410
1954	7,234	2,593	4,641	182	173	658	3,628	284
1955	5,515	2,076	3,439	164	77	279	2,919	263
1956	5,535	2,437	3,098	127	39	137	2,795	227
1957	5,452	2,185	3,267	108	47	114	2,998	180
1958	4,839	1,918	2,921	117	44	66	2,694	194
1959	5,215	2,641	2,574	98	26	33	2,417	199
1960	4,593	1,811	2,782	132	52	28	2,570	218
1961	4,388	1,627	2,761	218	44	18	2,481	346
1962	4,085	1,370	2,715	219	38	31	2,427	330
1963	4,140	434	3,706	367	52	42	3,245	410
1964	3,737	379	3,358	336	53	22	2,947	374
1965	3,505	410	3,095	329	52	39	2,675	373
1966	3,464	345	3,119	333	30	65	2,691	370

a Number less than one year of age estimated by assuming that states which did not report cases by age had the same age distribution of cases as states which did report by age.

Table A.I.17   Primary and secondary syphilis, number of cases and age-specific case rates per 100,000 population by age groups, color, and sex: United States, calendar years 1957, 1962 and 1965

Age	Year	Number of cases					Case rates				
		Total	White		Nonwhite		Total	White		Nonwhite	
			Male	Female	Male	Female		Male	Female	Male	Female
All ages	1957	6,581	1,787	604	2,426	1,764	3.9	2.4	.8	27.1	18.4
	1962	21,067	4,766	1,167	8,808	6,326	11.5	6.0	1.4	85.2	56.9
	1965	23,338	3,915	1,254	10,439	7,730	12.2	4.8	1.4	94.7	65.1
0-14	1957	121	17	10	20	74	.2	.1	0.0	.6	2.2
	1962	265	5	14	69	177	.5	0.0	.1	1.7	4.3
	1965	281	7	8	73	193	.5	0.0	0.0	1.6	4.4
15-19	1957	1,217	123	154	384	556	10.8	2.6	3.0	55.3	74.7
	1962	3,587	346	248	1,365	1,628	24.8	5.6	3.8	158.4	180.1
	1965	4,039	286	248	1,494	2,011	24.2	3.9	3.4	142.3	186.2
20-24	1957	1,896	448	144	759	545	19.8	12.1	3.1	137.5	81.3
	1962	6,063	1,046	310	2,697	2,010	55.8	24.1	6.0	435.7	271.6
	1965	6,575	918	354	3,032	2,271	52.5	18.3	5.9	426.4	273.3
25-29	1957	1,288	404	92	531	261	11.7	8.6	1.8	91.9	38.1
	1962	4,184	992	199	1,826	1,167	40.2	22.7	4.2	316.5	168.4
	1965	4,544	750	206	2,266	1,322	41.7	16.3	4.1	375.8	184.9
30-39	1957	1,299	474	100	494	231	5.5	4.6	.9	42.9	17.3
	1962	4,583	1,430	226	1,964	963	19.5	14.3	2.1	160.6	66.4
	1965	4,973	1,105	207	2,294	1,367	22.1	11.5	2.0	192.9	95.6
40-49	1957	482	200	51	165	66	2.2	2.1	.5	16.2	5.8
	1962	1,621	595	113	624	289	7.1	5.9	1.1	56.5	23.4
	1965	2,055	583	147	902	423	8.7	5.6	1.3	79.1	32.6
50 and over	1957	278	121	53	73	31	.7	.7	.3	4.9	1.9
	1962	764	352	57	263	92	1.8	1.9	.3	14.6	4.7
	1965	871	266	84	378	143	1.9	1.4	.4	20.1	6.8

Source: Venereal Disease Program, National Communicable Disease Center, Atlanta, Georgia.
Note: Cases not reported by age have been distributed by age on the basis of the known age distribution. Rates are based on population estimates of the Bureau of the Census. Numbers include Alaska and Hawaii for 1957, 1962 and 1965. Rates are based on cases excluding Alaska and Hawaii for 1957. For 1962 and 1965, rates are based on numbers for the United States, including Alaska and Hawaii.

Table A.I.18   Gonorrhea, number of cases and age-specific case rates per 100,000 population by age groups, color, and sex: United States, calendar years 1957, 1962 and 1965

Age	Year	Number of cases					Case rates				
		Total	White		Nonwhite		Total	White		Nonwhite	
			Male	Female	Male	Female		Male	Female	Male	Female
All ages	1957	214,872	31,340	12,622	118,537	52,373	127.6	42.9	16.4	1,324.9	546.0
	1962	263,714	52,046	20,057	139,515	52,096	143.5	65.9	24.1	1,349.7	468.8
	1965	324,925	64,714	25,164	180,498	54,549	169.3	78.7	29.0	1,636.7	459.2
0-14	1957	4,029	247	601	1,013	2,168	7.7	1.1	2.7	29.4	63.3
	1962	3,881	156	710	1,039	1,976	6.7	.6	2.9	25.0	47.7
	1965	4,525	298	741	1,274	2,212	7.6	1.1	3.0	28.6	49.9
15-19	1957	44,122	3,568	3,345	20,817	16,392	392.5	75.5	65.9	2,999.6	2,203.2
	1962	51,679	6,409	5,611	24,912	14,747	358.0	103.5	86.6	2,890.0	1,631.3
	1965	66,947	8,808	7,485	34,026	16,628	400.8	121.3	102.4	3,240.6	1,539.6
20-24	1957	70,831	9,471	3,561	40,782	17,017	738.1	255.8	76.2	7,388.0	2,539.9
	1962	91,591	17,675	6,602	49,580	17,734	842.3	407.7	127.5	8,009.2	2,396.5
	1965	114,945	23,178	8,847	64,123	18,797	918.5	461.8	148.6	9,018.7	2,262.0
25-29	1957	44,813	7,231	1,984	27,088	8,510	405.8	153.5	39.1	4,686.5	1,242.3
	1962	53,298	11,392	3,087	29,928	8,891	512.3	260.8	64.8	5,186.3	1,283.0
	1965	64,525	14,210	3,680	37,955	8,680	592.0	308.8	73.9	6,294.4	1,214.0
30-39	1957	38,908	7,029	2,061	23,220	6,598	163.4	68.5	18.6	2,015.6	494.2
	1962	46,153	10,973	2,746	25,788	6,646	196.6	109.4	25.5	2,108.6	458.0
	1965	52,588	11,927	2,843	31,563	6,255	234.0	123.8	27.8	2,654.6	437.4
40-49	1957	9,112	2,504	758	4,539	1,311	41.9	26.2	7.6	445.9	114.9
	1962	12,816	3,822	937	6,516	1,541	55.8	38.1	8.8	590.2	125.0
	1965	15,709	4,224	962	9,064	1,459	66.2	40.9	8.8	794.4	112.4
50 and over	1957	3,057	1,290	312	1,078	377	7.9	7.6	1.7	71.6	23.7
	1962	4,296	1,619	364	1,752	561	9.9	8.7	1.7	97.3	28.8
	1965	5,686	2,069	606	2,493	518	12.4	10.7	2.7	132.5	24.7

Note: Cases not reported by age have been distributed by age on the basis of the known age distribution. Rates are based on population estimates of the Bureau of the Census. Numbers include Alaska and Hawaii for 1957, 1962 and 1965. Rates are based on cases excluding Alaska and Hawaii for 1957. For 1962 and 1965, rates are based on numbers for the United States, including Alaska and Hawaii.

Appendix II
Mortality

Table A.II.1 Code numbers for syphilis and its sequelae according to successive International Statistical Classifications (ISC) of causes of death: United States, 1900-63

Cause of death	Revision of ISC and period in use						
	First 1900-09	Second 1910-20	Third [b] 1921-29	Fourth 1930-38	Fifth [c] 1939-48	Sixth 1949-57	Seventh 1958-63
Syphilis and its sequelae [a]	36,62,67	37,62,67	38,72,76 91a	34,80,83 96	30	020-029	020-029
Congenital syphilis	...	...	...	...	30f	020	020
Early syphilis	...	...	...	...		021	021
Aneurysm of aorta	...	...	91a	96	30d	022	022
Other cardiovascular syphilis					30e	023	023
Tabes dorsalis (locomotor ataxia)	62	52	72	80	30a	024	024
General paralysis of insane	67	67	76	83	30b	025	025
Other syphilis of central nervous system					30c	026	026
Other syphilis	36	37	38	34	30g	027-029	027-029

Source: National Center for Health Statistics; Vital Statistics Rates in the United States, 1900-1940(1943); Comparability Ratios: Mortality Statistics for the Fifth and Sixth Revisions: United States, (1950); Vital Statistics-Special Reports, vol. 51, no. 3, February 1964; Vital Statistics of the United States, vol. I, 1955 and 1958.

[a] Syphilis (all forms) includes aneurysm, except of heart, for 1921-38, inclusive; aneurysm of the aorta tabulated as syphilitic, except when the aneurysm was specified as nonsyphilitic in origin, 1935-55. Deaths from aneurysm of aorta tabulated as syphilitic only when specified as syphilitic in origin by the physician, 1955-63.

[b] In the Third Revision, 91a refers to ISC comparative designation for aneurysm of aorta due to syphilis.

[c] In the Fifth Revision, syphilis and its sequelae was assigned the ISC number 30 and subdivided a through g for other diseases caused by syphilis, i.e.: Locomotor ataxia (tabes dorsalis 30a; General paralysis 30b; Other syphilis of the central nervous system 30c; Aneurysm of the aorta 30d; Other syphilis of the circulatory system 30e; Congenital syphilis 30f; and Other and unspecified forms of syphilis 30g).

Table A.II.2 Comparability ratios for syphilis and its sequelae for Fifth and Sixth Revision of ISC; by color, sex, and age: United States (Sixth Revision ISC codes 020-029)

	All ages[a]	Under 1	1-4	5-14	15-24	25-34	35-44	45-54	55-64	65-74	75-84	85 and over
Total	.72	.97	*	*	.70	.69	.73	.74	.69	.69	.73	.64
Male	.72	.97	*	*	.79	.76	.72	.75	.69	.70	.73	.56
Female	.71	.97	*	*	.61	.61	.75	.73	.70	.67	.71	.75
White	.69	.95	*	*	.80	.60	.68	.69	.67	.69	.73	.63
Male	.69	.90	*	*	.79	.64	.65	.68	.67	.70	.73	.53
Female	.69	1.03	*	*	*	.57	.73	.70	.67	.66	.72	.76
Nonwhite	.77	.98	*	*	.56	.73	.76	.81	.76	.70	.72	*
Male	.78	1.03	*	*	*	.82	.77	.84	.75	.70	.75	*
Female	.74	.93	*	*	.46	.63	.76	.76	.78	.71	.66	*

Comparability ratios for other syphilitic conditions, total persons at all ages[a]

Condition	Comparability ratio
Congenital syphilis (020)	.95
Early syphilis (021)	No comparable category
Aneurysm of aorta (022)	.54
Other cardiovascular syphilis (023)	2.59
Tabes dorsalis (024)	.54
General paralysis of insane (025)	.66
Other syphilis of CNS (026)	.85
Other syphilis (027-029)	.14

Source: National Center for Health Statistics; Comparability Ratios Based on Mortality Statistics for the Fifth and Sixth Revisions; United States, (1950): Vital Statistics-Special Reports; vol. 51, no. 3, February, 1964; and Vital Statistics of the United States, 1949, Part I.

[a]Ratios for all ages include cases with age not stated.

Table A.II.3   Conditions coded as principal cause of death, with syphilis
and its sequelae as an associated cause: United States,
1955 (ISC codes 020-029)

Selected underlying cause of death	Certificates with syphilis reported as an associated cause	
	Number	Percent
Total conditions	2,910	
Excluding syphilis, coded both as underlying and associated cause	2,405	100.0
Diseases of circulatory system	1,087	45.2
Arteriosclerotic heart disease, including coronary disease	599	24.9
Other diseases of heart	391	16.3
Other diseases of circulatory system	97	4.0
Neoplasms	276	11.5
Diseases of the nervous system and sense organs	246	10.2
Diseases of the respiratory system	229	9.5
Pneumonia, except pneumonia of newborn	214	8.9
Infective and parasitic diseases (excluding syphilis)	126	5.2
Diseases of the digestive system	126	5.2
Diseases of genito-urinary system	45	1.9
Violent or accidental deaths	71	3.0
Other	199	8.2

Source: National Center for Health Statistics; Vital Statistics
of the United States: Supplement Multiple Cause of Death, 1955, (1965).

Table A.II.4   Estimated number of certificates with syphilis and its
               sequelae, reported as underlying cause and with any
               mention, by color and sex: United States, 1955

Cause of death	Total with mention	Coded as underlying cause	Ratio: total to underlying cause
Syphilis and its sequelae	6,735	3,825	1.76
White			
Male	3,535	1,834	1.93
Female	1,044	604	1.73
Nonwhite			
Male	1,571	1,006	1.56
Female	585	390	1.50
Congenital syphilis	73	51	1.43
Aneurysm of aorta	1,583	1,018	1.56
Other cardiovascular syphilis	2,048	1,600	1.28
Tabes dorsalis	261	131	1.99
Genereal paralysis of insane	1,131	464	2.44
Other syphilis of CNS	888	492	1.80
Other forms of late syphilis	184	39	4.72
Syphilis, unqualified	380	26	14.62
Other syphilis	187	4	---

Source: National Center for Health Statistics, Vital Statistics of
the United States: Supplement, Multiple Cause of Death, 1955, (1965).

Note: Changes in processing procedure produced a slight difference
in total deaths for syphilis. In the Supplement, Multiple Cause of Death,
1955, syphilis was coded as underlying cause of death 3,825 times and in
Vital Statistics of the United States, 1955, vols. I and II, syphilis was
coded as the underlying cause of death 3,834 times. For this reason, the
underlying cause of deaths by color-sex do not add to total on this table.

Table A.II.5 Deaths and death rates per 100,000 population for syphilis and its sequelae: United States, selected years from 1900 to 1965

Year	Deaths due to syphilis and its sequelae	Death rate			
		Syphilis and its sequelae	Tabes dorsalis	General paralysis of insane	Aneurysm of aorta
1965	2,434	1.3	0.0	0.0	0.8
1960	2,945	1.6	0.0	0.1	0.7
1955	3,834	2.3	0.1	0.3	0.7
1950	7,568	5.0	0.1	0.9	1.6
1945	14,062	10.6	0.4	3.3	2.2
1940	19,006	14.4	0.6	3.4	2.8
1939	19,604	15.0	0.6	3.4	3.0
1938	20,645	15.9	0.6	3.5	2.0
1937	20,802	16.1	0.7	3.2	2.0
1936	20,701	16.2	0.8	3.5	2.1
1935	19,560	15.4	0.7	3.6	1.9
1934	20,075	15.9	0.9	3.8	1.9
1933	18,984	15.1	0.9	3.6	1.8
1930	--	15.7	1.1	4.3	1.8
1925	--	17.3	1.6	5.8	1.8
1920	--	16.5	1.8	5.8	--
1915	--	17.7	2.6	7.5	--
1910	--	13.5	2.7	5.6	--
1900	--	12.0	2.0	7.4	--

Source: National Center for Health Statistics; Vital Statistics Rates in The United States, 1900-1940 and Vital Statistics of The United States (annual publications).

Note: Data before 1933 relate to the death registration states for the year specified; all data tabulated according to the revision of the ISC in effect in the year in which the death occurred. Deaths from aneurysm, except of heart, tabulated as syphilitic, 1921-38; deaths from aneurysm of the aorta tabulated as syphilitic, except when aneurysm specified as nonsyphilitic in origin, 1939-55; deaths from aneurysm of aorta tabulated as syphilitic only when specified as syphilitic in origin by the physician, 1955-65.

Table A.II.6   Death rates per 100,000 population for syphilis and its sequelae by age, total, both sexes: United States, selected years from 1900 to 1965

Year	All ages	Under 1	1-4	5-14	15-24	25-34	35-44	45-54	55-64	65-74	75-84	85 & over
1965	1.3	0.6	-	0.0*	0.0*	0.1	0.2	1.1	3.5	7.9	9.2	7.1
1960	1.6	0.7	-	0.0*	0.0*	0.2	0.5	1.9	5.6	9.1	8.7	9.5
1955	2.3	0.9	0.0*	0.0*	0.0*	0.2	1.0	4.0	7.9	11.7	10.8	7.2
1950	5.0	6.4	0.1*	0.0*	0.3	0.7	3.3	9.3	15.8	22.0	22.7	16.6
1949	5.8	9.5	0.1*	0.0*	0.3	0.9	4.1	11.1	18.6	22.9	23.1	20.8
1948	8.0	13.8	0.1*	0.1*	0.5	1.8	6.8	15.5	25.4	29.1	27.3	23.8
1945	10.6	27.8	0.4	0.2	1.3	4.2	11.8	20.3	29.3	30.3	26.5	25.4
1940	14.4	61.9	1.3	0.5	2.3	7.1	17.8	29.6	38.9	41.3	32.4	30.7
1939	15.0	64.1	1.7	0.5	2.5	8.1	19.0	29.6	41.0	41.5	37.3	30.1
1938	15.9	71.8	2.1	0.5	2.9	8.9	19.9	32.2	42.9	43.7	38.9	33.2
1937	16.1	77.8	1.9	0.6	2.6	9.1	21.2	32.9	43.5	43.5	40.0	34.5
1936	16.2	80.9	1.9	0.5	2.7	9.4	20.7	33.8	43.8	43.0	42.5	31.7
1935	15.4	76.5	1.9	0.6	2.9	9.0	20.8	32.9	40.3	39.1	37.1	41.1
1930	15.7	87.4	2.6	0.5	3.6	10.1	21.7	34.5	40.0	39.3	36.2	34.9
1925	17.3	84.8	2.8	0.6	3.3	10.0	27.5	39.1	42.4	46.0	42.5	41.6
1920	16.5	98.1	3.1	0.6	3.2	9.6	26.0	34.5	39.3	42.6	50.2	60.9
1919	16.2	102.9	3.2	0.6	3.1	9.6	24.7	33.6	37.7	42.1	48.5	63.9
1918	18.7	112.1	3.8	0.6	3.7	13.5	28.5	36.7	41.3	47.5	57.4	66.7
1917	19.1	131.7	4.5	0.6	3.2	11.7	28.8	37.3	43.9	51.7	57.7	73.4
1916	18.6	134.8	4.5	0.7	2.5	10.5	27.6	37.3	44.3	47.0	66.2	84.6
1915	17.7	129.0	3.5	0.5	2.0	9.9	26.5	33.9	40.9	49.5	72.1	76.0
1910	13.5	131.4	3.1	0.4	1.3	6.3	19.0	26.1	29.9	36.1	47.5	42.8
1905	13.8	---	---	---	---	---	---	---	---	---	---	---
1900	12.0	---	---	---	---	---	---	---	---	---	---	---

Source: National Center for Health Statistics, "Syphilis and its Sequelae," Vital Statistics-Special Reports, vol. 43, no. 3, May 15, 1956 and Vital Statistics of the United States, 1954-65.
Note: Data before 1935 relate to the death registration states; all data tabulated according to the revision cf the ISC in effect in the year in which death occurred. See text for qualification.

Table A.II.7   Deaths under one year of age and infant
mortality rates for syphilis and its
sequelae: United States, each geographic
division and state, 1939 and 1965
(ISC codes 020-029 for 1965; rates per
100,000 live births)

Geographic area	1965		1939	
	Deaths	Rate	Deaths	Rate
United States	25	.7	1,300	57.4
White male	7	.4	315	30.9
female	4	.3	248	25.7
Nonwhite male	7	2.2	424	295.3
female	7	2.2	313	224.6
New England	-	-	20	15.8
Connecticut	-	-	1	4.3
Maine	-	-	6	40.0
Massachusetts	-	-	7	11.0
New Hampshire	-	-	3	37.8
Rhode Island	-	-	1	9.6
Vermont	-	-	2	31.4
Middle Atlantic	3	.5	136	33.6
New Jersey	-	-	19	33.7
New York	3	.9	55	29.3
Pennsylvania	-	-	62	38.5
East North Central	4	.5	109	25.1
Illinois	1	.5	31	26.3
Indiana	-	-	20	34.3
Michigan	1	.6	22	23.3
Ohio	2	1.0	32	29.3
Wisconsin	-	-	4	7.4
West North Central	2	.7	72	31.4
Iowa	-	-	7	16.0
Kansas	-	-	8	27.5
Minnesota	-	-	11	21.9
Missouri	1	1.2	36	61.1
Nebraska	1	3.6	5	22.4
North Dakota	-	-	1	7.6
South Dakota	-	-	4	34.4
South Atlantic	2	.3	351	97.4
Delaware	-	-	5	114.1
District of Columbia	-	-	13	92.6
Florida	1	.9	54	167.0
Georgia	-	-	55	84.9
Maryland	-	-	20	70.7
North Carolina	1	1.0	66	83.4
South Carolina	-	-	53	123.8
Virginia	-	-	55	103.9
West Virginia	-	-	30	72.2

Table A.II.7 cont.

Geographic area	1965		1939	
	Deaths	Rate	Deaths	Rate
East South Central	3	1.2	225	99.1
Alabama	1	1.4	71	115.7
Kentucky	-	-	36	59.4
Mississippi	2	3.8	72	139.2
Tennessee	-	-	46	86.2
West South Central	9	2.4	284	114.1
Arkansas	-	-	34	95.6
Louisiana	1	1.3	106	217.0
Oklahoma	-	-	23	52.9
Texas	8	3.7	121	100.0
Mountain	-	-	57	65.0
Arizona	-	-	23	210.5
Colorado	-	-	5	24.2
Idaho	-	-	2	18.1
Montana	-	-	7	64.2
Nevada	-	-	-	-
New Mexico	-	-	19	133.7
Utah	-	-	-	-
Wyoming	-	-	1	20.4
Pacific	2	.4	46	31.4
Alaska	-	-	---	---
California	2	.6	42	40.6
Hawaii	-	-	---	---
Oregon	-	-	1	6.0
Washington	-	-	3	11.3

Table A.II.8   Death rates per 100,000 population for syphilis and its sequelae by age, color, and sex: United States, selected years from 1915 to 1965

Color, sex, year	All Ages	Under 1	1-4	5-14	15-24	25-34	35-44	45-54	55-64	65-74	75-84	85 & over
White male												
1965	1.5	0.4*	–	0.0*	0.0*	0.1*	0.2*	1.0	4.0	11.5	13.5	7.5
1960	1.9	0.6*	–	0.0*	0.0*	0.1*	0.4	1.6	6.4	12.6	11.7	10.0
1950	5.6	3.1	–	0.0*	0.2	0.3	1.9	8.0	19.6	31.3	30.9	18.8
1939	15.5	34.7	0.8	0.3	0.9	4.1	15.4	31.2	53.4	56.5	50.6	35.0
1938	16.3	41.6	1.1	0.4	1.0	4.8	16.4	34.2	55.5	57.4	50.8	34.7
1918	24.0	103.6	2.7	0.5	2.8	16.7	39.0	49.6	55.8	65.0	71.7	76.3
1917	24.0	---	---	---	---	---	---	---	---	---	---	---
1915	22.2	121.3	2.7	0.6	1.6	11.0	37.1	47.1	56.1	61.5	87.1	62.2
White female												
1965	0.6	0.3*	–	0.0*	0.0*	0.1*	0.1*	0.3	1.3	2.8	5.0	6.1
1960	0.7	0.2*	–	–	0.0*	0.0*	0.1*	0.5	1.8	3.1	4.7	7.0
1950	1.9	2.3	–	–	0.2*	0.2	1.1	2.7	4.7	8.3	12.0	13.4
1939	5.3	28.3	0.6	0.2*	1.2	2.7	5.6	9.0	13.2	16.0	18.0	20.0
1938	5.8	32.2	0.5*	0.2	1.4	3.2	5.8	10.2	14.6	17.3	21.8	21.7
1918	9.5	82.0	2.4	0.4	1.7	5.7	12.2	16.4	20.5	26.2	42.0	60.1
1917	10.1	---	---	---	---	---	---	---	---	---	---	---
1915	10.1	104.9	2.7	0.3*	1.3	5.6	10.6	15.1	19.8	33.1	58.8	90.5
Nonwhite male												
1965	4.0	2.2	–	0.0*	0.1*	0.9	1.5*	8.0	17.2	33.8	24.9	19.5*
1960	6.6	3.3*	–	0.0*	0.1*	0.7*	3.2	13.6	31.2	44.7	31.4	41.5*
1950	23.2	35.1	0.9*	0.2*	0.7*	5.9	25.4	69.1	90.3	84.5	74.3	42.9*
1939	74.5	354.0	8.3	1.8	10.2	59.8	132.1	183.7	192.7	158.2	164.1	77.6*
1938	77.6	376.5	11.4	2.1	12.9	61.9	133.0	188.2	197.8	188.2	158.3	120.3*
1918	54.2	360.5	18.3	3.1	19.7	56.8	75.9	97.4	117.9	103.6	144.9	93.2*
1917	57.7	---	---	---	---	---	---	---	---	---	---	---
1915	63.5	584.6	20.3	3.3*	17.1	48.0	87.5	98.2	153.4	153.1	102.4*	40.8*
Nonwhite female												
1965	1.7	2.2*	–	–	0.1*	0.3*	0.8*	2.7	7.8	11.7	11.0	5.6*
1960	2.6	1.6*	–	–	0.1*	0.7*	1.6*	6.2	12.4	12.4	13.1	12.4*
1950	9.4	27.5	0.3*	0.3*	0.9*	3.4	13.3	25.1	29.6	31.9	32.2	19.1*
1939	36.3	254.6	7.8	2.7	18.2	37.6	56.9	69.3	75.8	56.2	40.1	52.3*
1938	39.4	279.7	10.1	1.9	20.0	39.5	63.9	79.0	77.9	62.0	31.3*	59.1*
1918	31.7	330.8	21.2	2.8*	17.9	32.3	38.6	49.3	49.7	52.0	25.8*	39.9*
1917	30.5	---	---	---	---	---	---	---	---	---	---	---
1915	34.1	424.1	27.7	1.6*	10.8	30.7	41.0	50.9	44.4	78.8	26.5*	28.5*

Note: Data before 1940 relate to death registration states for the year specified; all data tabulated according to the revision of the ISC in effect in the year in which deaths occurred. See text for qualifications.

Table A.II.9 Age-adjusted death rates per 100,000 population for syphilis and its
sequelae, by color and sex: United States, 1910 to 1959-61

Year	Total			White			Nonwhite		
	Total	Male	Female	Total	Male	Female	Total	Male	Female
1959-61	1.4	2.2	0.7	1.0	1.6	0.5	5.3	7.5	3.4
1950	4.6	6.9	2.4	3.3	5.0	1.6	18.3	26.1	10.5
1949	5.3	7.9	2.8	3.7	5.7	1.7	21.7	30.4	13.0
1948	7.4	10.9	3.9	5.1	7.8	2.6	30.0	42.2	17.9
1945	9.8	14.7	5.0	6.7	10.3	3.1	39.9	57.6	22.4
1940	14.4	20.7	8.0	9.7	14.4	4.9	61.6	85.0	37.3
1939	15.1	21.5	8.6	10.3	15.3	5.2	62.5	84.0	40.0
1938	16.2	22.7	9.4	11.1	16.3	5.8	66.3	88.0	43.5
1937	16.6	23.3	9.6	11.5	16.9	6.0	66.4	88.5	43.0
1936	16.7	23.7	9.5	11.8	17.2	6.2	65.9	89.3	40.9
1935	16.0	22.6	9.2	11.4	16.6	6.0	62.5	84.0	39.6
1930	16.8	23.3	10.0	12.5	18.0	6.6	60.2	76.1	42.8
1925	18.7	26.3	10.6	15.4	22.3	8.1	57.3	72.9	39.6
1920	17.9	24.9	10.2	15.7	22.4	8.5	43.8	55.8	29.8
1919	17.5	24.0	10.5	15.6	21.8	9.0	39.2	49.0	28.0
1918	20.0	27.8	11.8	18.0	25.4	10.2	47.9	60.3	33.7
1917	20.5	28.3	12.1	---	---	---	---	---	---
1916	20.1	27.6	12.0	18.4	25.6	10.7	46.3	58.9	31.8
1915	19.1	25.9	11.7	17.7	24.1	10.7	52.5	67.1	35.1
1910	14.4	19.8	8.4	---	---	---	---	---	---

Source: National Center for Health Statistics, "Syphilis and Its Sequelae,"
Vital Statistics-Special Reports, vol. 43, no. 3, May 15, 1956, and Special
Tabulations for Monograph.
    Note: Data before 1935 relate to the death registration states for the
year specified; all data tabulated according to the revision of the ISC in
effect in the year in which death occurred. See text for qualification of data.

Table A.II.10 Deaths and death rates per 100,000 population for syphilis and its sequelae: United States, each geographic division and state, selected years from 1933 to 1965

Geographic area	Death rates					Deaths				
	1933	1939	1950	1960	1965	1933	1939	1950	1960	1965
United States	15.1	15.0	5.0	1.6	1.3	18,984	19,604	7,568	2,945	2,434
New England	10.2	9.9	3.9	1.6	1.4	841	830	367	172	161
Connecticut	12.9	10.8	4.5	1.5	1.0	209	184	90	38	28
Maine	8.9	8.7	3.7	0.8	0.8	72	73	36	8	8
Massachusetts	9.5	9.6	3.4	1.7	1.8	406	413	162	89	96
New Hampshire	8.1	11.7	5.8	3.1	1.5	38	57	28	17	10
Rhode Island	13.3	10.9	4.5	1.5	1.6	90	77	37	14	14
Vermont	7.3	7.3	3.7	2.3	1.3	26	26	14	10	5
Middle Atlantic	14.2	15.3	4.2	1.6	1.2	3,844	4,183	1,261	551	419
New Jersey	13.7	13.0	3.6	1.4	0.7	561	538	173	79	45
New York	15.1	16.5	4.7	1.4	1.0	1,972	2,204	691	226	176
Pennsylvania	13.4	14.6	3.8	2.1	1.7	1,311	1,441	397	238	198
East North Central	14.3	13.1	5.2	1.3	1.1	3,655	3,460	1,592	473	414
Illinois	14.5	12.9	4.9	0.9	1.1	1,121	1,010	436	85	114
Indiana	16.0	14.0	5.9	1.4	1.1	533	478	237	68	53
Michigan	13.1	13.1	5.2	1.1	1.1	628	674	329	92	87
Ohio	16.6	15.7	6.3	2.0	1.2	1,128	1,081	496	187	122
Wisconsin	8.1	7.0	2.9	0.9	0.9	245	217	94	33	38
West North Central	11.5	10.8	4.7	1.6	1.3	1,558	1,461	660	250	212
Iowa	10.5	7.9	4.0	1.2	0.9	261	200	106	37	25
Kansas	11.8	12.9	5.0	1.9	1.4	222	233	103	43	31
Minnesota	11.0	8.3	3.8	1.4	1.0	292	230	114	55	36
Missouri	16.5	16.8	7.0	2.3	2.1	613	632	264	94	93
Nebraska	8.3	6.8	2.7	1.4	1.0	114	90	37	17	15
North Dakota	4.2	5.6	3.4	0.5	1.1	28	36	20	4	7
South Dakota	4.1	6.2	2.6	1.2	0.7	28	40	16	9	5
South Atlantic	19.4	19.4	5.9	1.8	1.4	3,139	3,417	1,231	470	400
Delaware	19.4	17.0	3.5	1.3	1.8	48	45	11	9	9
District of Columbia	36.5	27.7	8.4	2.5	2.2	193	180	76	21	18
Florida	36.3	28.0	6.6	2.0	1.3	563	516	186	99	78
Georgia	17.3	20.4	5.9	1.7	1.2	518	633	203	73	54
Maryland	22.1	27.0	7.6	2.7	1.6	374	483	173	80	55

North Carolina	10.6	12.4	4.1	1.2	1.1	351	438	159	55	53
South Carolina	18.7	19.0	6.6	1.9	1.9	338	359	138	42	48
Virginia	20.1	17.9	5.6	1.5	1.3	506	474	184	60	57
West Virginia	13.7	15.3	5.4	1.9	1.5	248	289	101	35	28
East South Central	16.8	17.6	4.5	1.4	1.0	1,700	1,887	528	167	132
Alabama	18.4	20.7	5.4	1.6	1.1	499	582	171	53	39
Kentucky	13.4	11.9	3.1	1.4	1.4	356	335	90	40	43
Mississippi	15.0	24.3	5.5	1.5	1.3	411	528	120	30	30
Tennessee	15.9	15.3	4.3	1.1	0.5	434	442	147	43	20
West South Central	16.1	15.9	5.5	2.4	1.6	2,008	2,067	942	408	298
Arkansas	13.0	16.5	5.4	1.8	1.8	240	320	109	34	35
Louisiana	31.0	27.3	10.2	3.5	2.2	684	640	273	113	77
Oklahoma	9.9	11.8	5.3	1.8	1.3	238	276	113	41	33
Texas	14.1	13.0	5.3	2.3	1.4	846	831	447	222	153
Mountain	11.5	13.7	4.7	1.4	1.2	438	563	241	98	97
Arizona	15.6	22.5	6.1	1.8	0.8	71	111	47	27	13
Colorado	12.8	14.6	3.7	1.9	1.1	135	162	55	32	22
Idaho	6.6	9.5	3.7	1.0	1.6	30	49	21	6	11
Montana	11.1	13.2	5.2	1.0	1.0	59	73	30	5	7
Nevada	14.4	12.9	9.4	2.5	2.0	14	14	14	8	7
New Mexico	14.6	17.3	6.0	1.2	1.3	66	90	40	13	13
Utah	6.3	5.3	3.8	0.7	1.3	33	29	23	6	13
Wyoming	13.1	14.3	3.3	0.9	2.6	30	35	11	4	9
Pacific	21.1	18.1	5.1	1.7	1.2	1,801	1,736	746	356	301
Alaska	--	--	--	--	-	--	--	--	-	-
California	22.9	19.5	5.5	1.7	1.2	1,366	1,320	589	256	230
Hawaii	--	--	--	0.3	0.7	--	--	--	5	5
Oregon	18.4	14.8	4.3	1.8	0.3	180	159	69	31	16
Washington	16.3	15.0	3.8	1.9	1.7	255	257	88	59	50

Note: Syphilis (all forms) includes "Aneurysm (except of heart)" 1933–1938; aneurysm of aorta tabulated as syphilitic, except when aneurysm was specified as nonsyphilitic in origin, 1939–1955; aneurysm of aorta tabulated as syphilitic only when specified as syphilitic in origin by the physician, 1955–1963. Deaths tabulated by place of occurrence prior to 1942, and by place of residence since then. Data tabulated according to the revision of the ISC in effect in the year in which death occurred.

Table A.II.11 Death and death rates per 100,000 population for syphilis and its
sequelae by age, color, and sex: United States, 1959-61
(ISC codes 020-029)

Age	Death rate					Deaths				
		White		Nonwhite			White		Nonwhite	
	Total	Male	Female	Male	Female	Total	Male	Female	Male	Female
All ages						8,869	4,426	1,592	1,931	920
Crude death rate	1.6	1.9	0.7	6.5	2.9					
Age-adjusted death rate	1.4	1.6	0.5	7.5	3.4					
Under 1	0.6	0.4	0.2	2.9	1.4	71	20	11	27	13
1 - 4	0.0	-	-	-	0.1	2	-	-	-	2
5 - 14	0.0	0.0	0.0	0.0	0.0	8	3	2	2	1
15 - 24	0.0	0.0	0.0	0.1	0.1	29	12	7	6	4
25 - 34	0.2	0.1	0.1	0.7	0.5	107	40	20	25	22
35 - 44	0.5	0.4	0.1	3.6	1.7	355	112	46	129	68
45 - 54	2.0	1.5	0.6	14.3	7.3	1,218	415	159	420	224
55 - 64	5.6	6.5	1.6	31.2	14.0	2,630	1,335	355	643	297
65 - 74	8.9	12.2	3.2	40.0	14.4	2,933	1,725	517	496	195
75 - 84	9.0	11.6	5.1	31.6	16.3	1,250	650	376	142	82
85 & over	9.2	11.0	6.3	39.3	9.1	256	109	99	37	11
65 & over						4,439	2,484	992	675	288
Crude death rate	8.9	12.0	3.9	37.8	14.5					
Age-adjusted death rate	8.9	12.0	3.8	37.8	14.7					

Table A.II.12 Deaths for all ages and for ages 65 and over by color and sex for syphilis and its sequelae: United States, each geographic division and state, 1959-61 (ISC codes 020-029)

Geographic area	All ages					Ages 65 and over				
		White		Nonwhite			White		Nonwhite	
	Total	Male	Female	Male	Female	Total	Male	Female	Male	Female
United States	8,869	4,426	1,592	1,931	920	4,439	2,484	992	675	288
New England	501	338	131	22	10	322	210	97	10	5
Connecticut	104	62	28	9	5	66	42	17	4	3
Maine	37	24	12	1	-	23	13	10	-	1
Massachusetts	260	179	67	11	3	175	115	53	6	1
New Hampshire	41	28	13	-	-	23	14	9	-	-
Rhode Island	36	25	8	1	2	21	14	6	-	1
Vermont	23	20	3	-	-	14	12	2	-	-
Middle Atlantic	1,663	889	330	287	157	858	505	203	94	56
New Jersey	251	143	42	38	28	130	80	28	12	10
New York	679	373	127	119	60	355	220	83	35	17
Pennsylvania	733	373	161	130	69	373	205	92	47	29
East North Central	1,484	798	304	253	129	753	439	184	90	40
Illinois	260	135	51	55	19	133	78	31	20	4
Indiana	225	135	57	23	10	130	78	38	9	5
Michigan	266	135	51	57	23	127	73	29	19	6
Ohio	621	307	125	115	74	300	163	71	41	25
Wisconsin	112	86	20	3	3	63	47	15	1	-
West North Central	714	433	167	86	28	410	246	108	44	12
Iowa	107	65	39	3	-	68	38	28	2	-
Kansas	118	70	26	12	10	65	41	14	4	6
Minnesota	135	104	28	2	1	81	58	20	2	1
Missouri	275	143	54	62	16	147	77	34	31	5
Nebraska	40	24	9	6	1	21	12	4	5	-
North Dakota	12	9	3	-	-	9	6	3	-	-
South Dakota	27	18	8	1	-	19	14	5	-	-
South Atlantic	1,470	464	182	557	267	585	244	112	162	67
Delaware	26	11	5	4	6	7	4	-	1	2
District of Columbia	55	6	8	25	16	25	1	7	10	7

Table A.II.12 cont.

Geographic area	All ages					Ages 65 and over				
		White		Nonwhite			White		Nonwhite	
	Total	Male	Female	Male	Female	Total	Male	Female	Male	Female
Florida	300	102	42	104	52	124	65	32	18	9
Georgia	237	55	10	120	52	85	29	3	43	10
Maryland	259	84	28	98	49	105	37	19	32	17
North Carolina	156	55	23	52	26	62	27	13	16	6
South Carolina	144	38	17	67	22	49	22	10	12	5
Virginia	188	56	24	69	39	74	30	14	19	11
West Virginia	105	57	25	18	5	54	29	14	11	-
East South Central	558	188	55	205	110	219	76	27	76	40
Alabama	184	42	10	78	54	75	17	6	31	21
Kentucky	142	77	28	26	11	57	27	13	13	4
Mississippi	112	18	5	60	29	46	11	2	21	12
Tennessee	120	51	12	41	16	41	21	6	11	3
West South Central	1,122	452	132	377	161	513	244	82	141	46
Arkansas	100	43	9	34	14	54	26	7	18	3
Louisiana	338	56	22	177	83	135	30	15	64	26
Oklahoma	119	80	18	12	9	65	45	12	5	3
Texas	565	273	83	154	55	259	143	48	54	14
Mountain	290	183	73	26	8	180	116	45	13	6
Arizona	56	33	10	11	2	30	19	7	3	1
Colorado	88	46	32	7	3	57	30	20	4	3
Idaho	24	19	5	-	-	19	15	4	-	-
Montana	30	23	6	1	-	22	17	4	1	-
Nevada	20	14	4	2	-	12	10	1	1	-
New Mexico	34	19	10	2	3	18	8	6	2	2
Utah	22	17	2	2	-	10	8	0	2	-
Wyoming	16	12	4	-	-	12	9	3	-	-
Pacific	1,067	681	218	118	50	599	404	134	45	16
Alaska	2	-	-	1	1	-	-	-	-	-
California	815	515	165	97	38	444	300	98	35	11
Hawaii	15	2	2	7	4	6	-	-	4	2
Oregon	72	48	13	8	3	39	26	9	3	1
Washington	163	116	38	5	4	110	78	27	3	2

Age-adjusted death rates per 100,000 population for all ages and for ages 65 and over by color and sex for syphilis and its sequelae: United States, each geographic division and state, 1959-61 (ISC codes 020-029)

Geographic area	All ages					Ages 65 and over				
	Total	White Male	White Female	Nonwhite Male	Nonwhite Female	Total	White Male	White Female	Nonwhite Male	Nonwhite Female
United States	1.4	1.6	0.5	7.5	3.4	8.9	12.0	3.8	37.8	14.7
New England	1.2	1.8	0.5	7.3	3.2*	9.5	14.8	4.8	48.8*	22.2*
Connecticut	1.1	1.4	0.5	8.4*	4.5*	9.0	13.4	4.1*	67.2*	42.0*
Maine	1.0	1.4	0.5*	24.9*	-	6.8	9.0*	5.1*	-	-
Massachusetts	1.2	1.9	0.5	6.9*	1.8*	10.0	16.3	5.0	51.6*	6.9*
New Hampshire	1.7	2.5	1.0*	-	-	11.3	16.0*	7.4*	-	-
Rhode Island	1.1	1.6	0.4*	4.6*	9.1*	8.0	12.5*	4.0*	-	59.5*
Vermont	1.5	2.8	0.3*	-	-	10.5*	21.0*	2.3*	-	-
Middle Atlantic	1.3	1.5	0.5	8.1	4.0	8.4	11.7	3.7	46.0	23.3
New Jersey	1.1	1.5	0.4	6.2	4.1	7.7	11.4	2.9	32.3*	22.9*
New York	1.0	1.2	0.7	6.9	2.9	7.0	10.2	3.0	38.1	14.8*
Pennsylvania	1.7	1.9	0.7	11.0	5.6	11.0	14.2	5.1	63.0	35.7
East North Central	1.1	1.4	0.5	7.0	3.4	7.5	10.1	3.4	41.3	16.9
Illinois	0.7	0.8	0.3	4.4	1.4*	4.6	6.4	2.0	26.0	4.7*
Indiana	1.3	1.8	0.6	6.4	2.8*	9.6	13.6	5.2	36.6*	20.4*
Michigan	1.0	1.1	0.4	6.6	2.5	6.6	8.5	2.8	39.9*	12.0*
Ohio	1.9	2.0	0.7	11.2	7.1	11.1	14.2	4.9	63.4	35.8
Wisconsin	0.8	1.2	0.2	3.7*	3.7*	5.2	8.4	2.2*	21.1*	-
West North Central	1.2	1.6	0.5	9.4	3.0	8.0	10.8	3.8	63.2	16.2*
Iowa	0.9	1.2	0.6	6.7*	-	6.8	8.7	5.0	61.9*	-
Kansas	1.4	1.9	0.6	8.6*	6.2*	9.0	13.3	3.1	32.1*	45.8*
Minnesota	1.0	1.7	0.4	3.7*	2.1*	7.7	11.6	3.6	53.9*	30.4*
Missouri	1.6	1.9	0.6	10.6	2.6*	10.1	12.7	4.1	70.4	10.5*
Nebraska	0.7	0.9	0.3*	12.4*	2.6*	4.3	5.2*	1.5*	146.6*	-
North Dakota	0.5*	0.8*	0.2*	-	-	5.4*	7.4*	3.6*	-	-
South Dakota	1.0	1.3*	0.7*	3.3*	-	8.6*	13.3*	4.2*	-	-
South Atlantic	1.8	1.5	0.5	8.0	3.5	9.3	10.3	3.7	33.9	11.9
Delaware	1.9	1.9*	0.9*	4.1*	7.7*	6.5*	9.4*	-	17.5*	37.4*
District of Columbia	1.9	0.9*	0.7*	5.4	2.9*	11.8	1.8*	7.8*	37.5*	19.8*

Table A.II.13 cont.

Geographic area	All ages					Ages 65 and over				
		White		Nonwhite			White		Nonwhite	
	Total	Male	Female	Male	Female	Total	Male	Female	Male	Female
Florida	1.6	1.2	0.4	9.7	4.7	7.4	8.7	4.1	27.2*	12.7*
Georgia	2.1	1.4	0.2*	9.2	3.3	9.8	10.6	0.7*	44.6	7.6*
Maryland	2.8	2.3	0.6	15.2	7.7	15.5	14.7	5.3*	79.9	40.8*
North Carolina	1.2	1.2	0.4	4.1	1.9	6.6	8.1	3.1*	18.6*	6.0*
South Carolina	2.3	2.0	0.7*	8.1	2.2	10.9	16.9	5.1*	19.1*	6.2*
Virginia	1.6	1.2	0.4	6.6	3.5	8.5	9.8	3.4*	24.6*	12.7*
West Virginia	1.6	1.9	0.8	9.6*	3.3*	10.3	12.2	5.4*	77.2*	-
East South Central	1.4	1.3	0.3	5.6	2.7	7.0	6.8	1.9	24.9	11.8
Alabama	1.8	1.2	0.2*	6.2	3.7	9.6	7.0*	1.7*	30.6	17.3
Kentucky	1.4	1.7	0.6	6.9	3.2*	6.6	7.3	2.9*	41.7*	11.5*
Mississippi	1.6	0.8*	0.2*	4.9	2.1	8.1	6.9*	1.0*	19.4	10.9*
Tennessee	1.1	1.1	0.2*	5.0	1.8*	4.6	6.2	1.5*	17.1*	4.1*
West South Central	2.0	2.0	0.5	9.8	3.9	12.0	14.8	4.1	44.8	13.3
Arkansas	1.4	1.5	0.3*	5.4	2.1*	9.5	11.7	2.9*	32.0*	5.3*
Louisiana	3.5	1.8	0.6	13.5	5.7	18.7	13.8	5.6*	60.5	21.1
Oklahoma	1.3	2.0	0.4*	3.7*	2.3*	8.5	14.2	2.7*	18.3*	10.8*
Texas	1.9	2.2	0.6	9.5	3.2	11.6	16.0	4.4	43.4	10.4*
Mountain	1.4	1.8	0.7	6.5	2.6*	11.3	15.6	5.5	49.6*	28.7*
Arizona	1.5	1.9	0.6*	6.6*	1.8*	11.1	15.1*	5.5*	29.3*	13.0*
Colorado	1.4	1.6	1.0	11.7*	4.4*	11.7	14.1	7.1	88.8*	64.1*
Idaho	1.0	1.6*	0.4*	-	-	11.1*	17.6*	4.6*	-	-
Montana	1.2	1.8	0.5*	2.8*	-	11.2	17.1*	4.4*	41.3*	-
Nevada	2.4	3.3*	1.2*	9.2*	-	22.1*	35.6*	4.4*	75.8*	-
New Mexico	1.5	1.8*	1.0*	2.9*	5.8*	11.9*	11.2*	8.5*	43.0*	58.3*
Utah	0.9	1.5*	0.2*	9.4*	-	5.7*	9.9*	-	113.4*	-
Wyoming	1.4*	2.1*	0.8*	-	-	14.9*	22.1*	7.7*	-	-
Pacific	1.4	2.1	0.6	5.0	2.5	10.6	16.8	4.3	32.0	13.5*
Alaska	0.4*	-	-	2.0*	2.6*	-	-	-	-	-
California	1.5	2.2	0.6	6.4	2.7	10.7	17.3	4.2	39.6	13.7*
Hawaii	1.1*	1.1*	1.1*	1.2*	1.0*	6.9*	-	-	10.6*	7.4*
Oregon	1.0	1.4	0.3*	15.3*	7.7*	6.9	10.0	2.9*	76.8*	45.0*
Washington	1.5	2.3	0.7	4.0*	4.6*	13.2	20.4	5.8	35.9*	34.2*

Table A.II.14   Death rates per 100,000 population for syphilis and its sequelae by color and sex, age-adjusted for all ages for metropolitan and non-metropolitan counties in each geographic division: United States, 1959-61 (ISC codes 020-029)

Sex; geographic division	White				Nonwhite		
	Metropolitan counties			Non-metro-politan counties	Metropolitan counties		Non-metro-politan counties
	Total	with central city	without central city		Total	without central city	
Male							
United States	1.7	1.8	1.5*	1.4	8.5	8.0	5.8*
New England	1.7*	1.8*	1.6*	1.9*	6.6*	0.0*	16.6*
Middle Atlantic	1.5	1.6*	1.3*	1.5*	8.3*	8.3	6.1*
East North Central	1.4*	1.4*	1.2*	1.4*	7.1*	2.8*	5.9*
West North Central	2.3*	2.5*	1.4*	1.1*	9.3*	9.9*	9.6*
South Atlantic	1.6*	1.7*	1.5*	1.3*	9.7*	9.0	6.5*
East South Central	1.8*	1.7*	2.7*	1.1*	7.6*	8.8*	4.3*
West South Central	2.3*	2.4*	1.5*	1.8*	13.8*	9.9*	6.6*
Mountain	1.9*	1.9*	1.2*	1.8*	8.8*	0.0*	4.7*
Pacific	2.1*	2.1*	2.1*	2.2*	5.6*	9.2*	2.7*
Female							
United States	0.5	0.5*	0.5*	0.5*	3.7*	5.6	2.7*
New England	0.5*	0.5*	0.7*	0.5*	3.5*	16.5*	0.0*
Middle Atlantic	0.5*	0.5*	0.4*	0.5*	4.0*	3.9	4.0*
East North Central	0.5*	0.5*	0.5*	0.5*	3.3*	5.1*	4.9*
West North Central	0.6*	0.6*	0.3*	0.5*	3.1*	4.6*	2.3*
South Atlantic	0.5*	0.5*	0.4*	0.5*	4.7*	8.3	2.4*
East South Central	0.5*	0.4*	1.0*	0.2*	3.0*	6.2*	2.5*
West South Central	0.6*	0.5*	0.8*	0.5*	4.9*	5.9*	2.9*
Mountain	0.7*	0.7*	0.7*	0.7*	2.2*	0.0*	3.1*
Pacific	0.5*	0.5*	0.6*	0.7*	2.3*	6.5*	3.6*

202

Table A.II.15 Age-adjusted death rates per 100,000 population for syphilis and its sequelae by marital status, color, and sex: United States for ages 15 and over, 15-64, and 65 and over; geographic divisions for ages 15-64 only, 1959-61 (ISC codes 020-029)

Sex, age, area	White				Nonwhite			
	Single	Married	Widowed	Divorced	Single	Married	Widowed	Divorced
Male								
United States								
15 and over	3.4*	1.8	3.3*	6.3*	14.1*	7.9	16.5*	22.5*
15-64	1.9*	0.9	2.1*	4.2*	10.1*	5.5	13.8*	14.9*
65 and over	18.5	10.5	15.1	26.5	53.1*	31.8	42.8	97.8*
15-64								
New England	1.8*	0.9*	2.0*	2.7*	9.9*	4.6*	5.5*	11.6*
Middle Atlantic	1.8*	0.9*	1.5*	4.2*	9.1*	5.2*	21.7*	13.9*
East North Central	1.7*	0.8*	1.5*	5.1*	6.7*	5.4*	6.7*	12.7*
West North Central	2.4*	0.8*	2.1*	6.8*	15.6*	4.6*	15.3*	13.0*
South Atlantic	1.9*	0.9*	2.3*	2.7*	13.5*	6.4*	14.1*	16.4*
East South Central	2.0*	1.0*	2.6*	4.2*	8.8*	4.9*	8.6*	9.8*
West South Central	2.2*	1.1*	2.4*	5.5*	17.4*	7.1	23.7*	26.7*
Mountain	1.4*	0.9*	4.5*	1.5*	13.2*	2.8*	4.6*	10.5*
Pacific	2.2*	1.0*	3.2*	3.9*	4.1*	3.2*	5.6*	12.2*
Female								
United States								
15 and over	0.6*	0.6	0.8*	1.5*	7.0*	3.0	5.9*	5.8*
15-64	0.5*	0.3	0.5*	0.8*	5.9*	2.2	5.0*	4.5*
65 and over	2.2*	3.6	4.2	7.7*	18.2*	10.8*	15.1	18.9*
15-64								
New England	0.4*	0.3*	0.4*	0.2*	-	2.2*	3.6*	-
Middle Atlantic	0.3*	0.3*	0.3*	0.8*	4.8*	2.3*	5.1*	4.6*
East North Central	0.8*	0.2*	0.4*	1.0*	4.2*	2.6*	4.3*	3.4*
West North Central	1.0*	0.2*	0.7*	0.8*	-	1.8*	4.2*	4.2*
South Atlantic	0.2*	0.3*	0.5*	0.5*	8.0*	2.5*	5.5*	3.5*
East South Central	0.3*	0.2*	0.5*	1.3*	4.4*	1.8*	3.1*	4.3*
West South Central	0.4*	0.2*	0.3*	1.2*	11.8*	2.2*	7.3*	7.9*
Mountain	0.8*	0.4*	0.3*	1.6*	-	0.7*	1.8*	-
Pacific	0.4*	0.4*	1.1*	0.7*	1.1*	1.5*	3.9*	4.2*

Table A.II.16   Age-adjusted death rates per 100,000 population for syphilis and its sequelae for the white native-born and white foreign-born by sex, for all ages, under 65 years, and 65 and over in each geographic division: United States, 1959-61 (ISC codes 020-029)

Nativity; sex; age	New England	Middle Atlantic	East North Central	West North Central	South Atlantic	East South Central	West South Central	Mountain	Pacific
White native born									
Male									
All ages	1.8*	1.6*	1.4*	1.5*	1.4*	1.3*	1.9*	1.7*	2.1*
Under 65	0.9*	0.8	0.7*	0.8*	0.7*	0.9*	1.0*	0.8*	1.0*
65 and over	14.2	12.7	10.6	10.7	10.3	7.0*	14.7	13.5*	17.1
Female									
All ages	0.5*	0.5*	0.5*	0.5*	0.5*	0.3*	0.5*	0.7*	0.6*
Under 65	0.1*	0.2*	0.3*	0.3*	0.3*	0.2*	0.2*	0.4*	0.3*
65 and over	5.5*	4.3	3.6	3.7	3.7	1.8*	4.2	5.2*	4.1
White foreign born									
Male									
All ages	1.5*	1.5*	1.2*	2.4*	1.8*	3.1*	4.7*	2.7*	2.2*
Under 65	0.5*	0.8*	0.6*	1.6*	1.0*	2.9*	3.6*	0.8*	1.1*
65 and over	15.5	10.6	9.1	13.1*	12.6*	5.9*	19.6*	28.6*	17.1
Female									
All ages	0.6*	0.3*	0.5*	0.6*	0.6*	0.5*	1.2*	0.7*	0.6*
Under 65	0.4*	0.1*	0.3*	0.3*	0.3*	0.0*	1.1*	0.2*	0.3*
65 and over	3.7*	2.5*	2.7	4.2*	4.8*	7.1*	2.3*	7.8*	5.2*

Table A.II.17 Deaths and death rates per 100,000 population for syphilis and its sequelae (category numbers 020-029, Seventh Revision of the International Lists, 1955) by color and sex: United States death registration states, selected years

Sex; color	1965	1964	1961	1960	1955	1950	1945	1940	1935	1930	1920	1910	1900
Deaths													
Total	2,434	2,619	2,850	2,945	3,834	7,568	14,062	19,006	19,560	---	---	---	---
Male	1,732	1,829	2,032	2,145	2,840	5,550	10,402	13,760	14,001	---	---	---	---
Female	702	790	818	800	994	2,018	3,660	5,246	5,559	---	---	---	---
White	1,789	1,889	1,892	2,019	2,438	5,024	8,892	11,701	12,554	---	---	---	---
Male	1,288	1,344	1,405	1,492	1,834	3,764	6,765	8,768	9,301	---	---	---	---
Female	501	545	487	527	604	1,260	2,127	2,933	3,253	---	---	---	---
Nonwhite	645	730	958	926	1,396	2,544	5,170	7,305	7,006	---	---	---	---
Male	444	485	627	653	1,006	1,786	3,637	4,992	4,700	---	---	---	---
Female	201	248	331	273	390	758	1,533	2,313	2,306	---	---	---	---
Death rate													
Total	1.3	1.4	1.6	1.6	2.3	5.0	10.7	14.4	15.4	15.7	16.5	13.5	12.0
Male	1.8	1.9	2.3	2.4	3.5	7.4	16.6	20.8	21.8	21.9	23.1	18.4	15.6
Female	0.7	0.8	0.9	0.9	1.2	2.7	5.2	8.0	8.8	9.5	9.7	8.3	8.4
White	1.0	1.1	1.2	1.3	1.7	3.7	7.5	9.9	11.0	11.7	14.5	13.0	---
Male	1.5	1.6	1.8	1.9	2.5	5.6	12.1	14.7	16.1	17.0	20.7	17.9	---
Female	0.6	0.6	0.6	0.7	0.8	1.9	3.4	5.0	5.8	6.2	8.0	7.9	---
Nonwhite	2.8	3.2	4.5	4.5	7.9	16.1	36.8	54.3	54.0	52.5	38.8	30.8	---
Male	4.0	4.4	6.1	6.6	11.6	23.2	54.4	75.5	73.3	67.0	49.7	36.1	---
Female	1.7	2.1	3.1	2.6	4.3	9.4	20.8	33.8	35.2	38.1	27.7	24.7	---

(The number of death-registration states increased to the entire United States in 1933.)

Note: Data tabulated according to the revision of the ISC in effect in the year in which the deaths occurred. Aneurysm, except of heart, tabulated for 1921-38. Prior to 1939, aneurysm had little weight in the Manual of Joint Causes of Death and was frequently tabulated under associated causes. Deaths for aneurysm of the aorta tabulated as syphilitic, except when the aneurysm was specified as nonsyphilitic in origin, 1939-55; deaths from aneurysm of aorta tabulated as syphilitic only when specified as syphilitic in origin by the physician, 1955-65.

Table A.II.18 Deaths and death rates per 100,000 population for aneurysm of aorta, other cardiovascular syphilis, tabes dorsalis, and general paralysis of the insane by color and sex: United States, selected years from 1900 to 1965

Cause of death; year	Death rate					Deaths				
	Total	White Male	White Female	Nonwhite Male	Nonwhite Female	Total	White Male	White Female	Nonwhite Male	Nonwhite Female
Aneurysm of aorta[a] (Code 022)										
1965	0.8	1.1	0.4	1.6	0.7	1,504	903	342	176	83
1960	0.7	1.0	0.3	1.8	0.8	1,337	801	275	176	85
1955	0.7	0.8	0.3	2.4	0.9	1,127	615	217	209	86
1950	1.6	2.2	0.7	4.4	1.9	2,377	1,444	441	341	151
1945	2.2	3.0	0.7	9.3	2.4	2,904	1,668	440	621	175
1940	2.8	3.4	0.9	12.8	3.7	3,635	2,022	512	846	255
1935	1.9	2.5	0.9	5.8	2.4	2,440	1,430	484	368	158
1930	1.8	--	--	--	--	--	--	--	--	--
Other cardio-vascular syphilis (Code 023)										
1965	0.3	0.3	0.1	1.7	0.6	549	213	75	186	75
1960	0.6	0.5	0.2	3.3	1.2	1,002	385	162	328	127
1955	0.9	0.9	0.3	5.7	2.1	1,545	668	193	491	193
1950	1.6	1.6	0.5	8.9	3.2	2,351	1,086	327	682	256
1945	0.8	0.8	0.1	5.4	1.5	1,006	447	90	358	111
1940	1.2	1.0	0.2	8.9	2.8	1,525	606	141	588	190
Tabes dorsalis (Code 024)										
1965	0.0	0.0	0.0	--	0.0	43	31	11	-	1
1960	0.0	0.1	0.0	0.1	0.0	62	41	9	8	4
1955	0.1	0.1	0.0	0.2	0.0	110	75	15	17	3

Table A.II.18 cont.

Cause of death; year	Death rate					Deaths				
	Total	White		Nonwhite		Total	White		Nonwhite	
		Male	Female	Male	Female		Male	Female	Male	Female
1950	0.1	0.2	0.0	0.2	0.1	174	119	29	17	9
1945	0.4	0.6	0.1	0.7	0.3	507	355	88	44	20
1940	0.6	0.9	0.2	1.1	0.1	740	525	133	72	10
1935	0.7	1.2	0.3	1.0	0.3	942	692	163	66	21
1930	1.1	--	--	--	--	--	--	--	--	--
1920	1.8	--	--	--	--	--	--	--	--	--
1910	2.7	--	--	--	--	--	--	--	--	--
1900	2.0	--	--	--	--	--	--	--	--	--
General paralysis of the insane (Code 025)										
1965	0.0	0.1	0.0	0.2	0.1	96	45	24	21	6
1960	0.1	0.1	0.0	0.5	0.2	204	102	35	48	19
1955	0.3	0.3	0.1	1.7	0.3	464	211	79	147	27
1950	0.9	0.9	0.3	5.2	1.4	1,301	576	209	401	115
1945	3.3	3.9	1.0	18.1	4.7	4,374	2,180	642	1,207	345
1940	3.4	4.0	1.2	15.7	4.3	4,423	2,404	687	1,036	296
1935	3.6	4.6	1.5	13.6	3.6	4,588	2,656	823	872	237
1930	4.1	5.6	1.5	11.7	4.5	--	--	--	--	--
1920	5.8	8.5	2.9	9.1	3.5	--	--	--	--	--
1910	5.6	--	--	--	--	--	--	--	--	--
1900	7.4	--	--	--	--	--	--	--	--	--

Note: Since data before 1933 relate to the death registration states for the year specified, the numbers of deaths for these years are not shown. Data tabulated according to the revision of the ISC in effect in the year in which death occurred.

a Aneurysm, except of heart, tabulated for 1921-38. Prior to 1939, aneurysm had little weight in the Manual of Joint Causes of Death and was frequently tabulated under associated causes. Deaths for aneurysm of the aorta tabulated as syphilitic, except when the aneurysm was specified as nonsyphilitic in origin, 1939-55. Deaths from aneurysm of aorta tabulated as syphilitic only when specified as syphilitic in origin by the physician, 1955-65.

Table A.II.19   Deaths and death rates per 100,000 population for aneurysm of aorta
and other cardiovascular syphilis by age, color, and sex: United States,
1959-61 (ISC codes 022-023)

Age	Death rate					Deaths				
		White		Nonwhite			White		Nonwhite	
	Total	Male	Female	Male	Female	Total	Male	Female	Male	Female
All ages						6,946	3,510	1,231	1,488	717
Crude death rate	1.3	1.5	0.5	5.0	2.3					
Age-adjusted death rate	1.1	1.3	0.4	5.8	2.6					
Under 1	-	-	-	-	-	-	-	-	-	-
1 - 4	-	-	-	-	-	-	-	-	-	-
5 - 14	0.0	0.0	-	-	-	1	1	-	-	-
15 - 24	0.0	0.0	0.0	0.0	-	16	11	3	2	-
25 - 34	0.1	0.1	0.0	0.5	0.3	74	30	11	18	15
35 - 44	0.4	0.3	0.1	2.4	1.2	253	95	24	86	48
45 - 54	1.5	1.1	.4	11.1	5.7	911	302	105	327	177
55 - 64	4.4	5.0	1.2	24.7	11.3	2,048	1,030	269	508	241
65 - 74	7.2	9.9	2.5	32.1	12.1	2,372	1,397	411	399	165
75 - 84	7.5	9.7	4.4	25.4	12.3	1,040	543	321	114	62
85 & over	8.0	9.8	5.5	31.9	7.4	223	97	87	30	9
65 & over						3,635	2,037	819	543	236
Crude death rate	7.3	9.8	3.3	30.4	11.9					
Age-adjusted death rate	7.3	9.8	3.1	30.4	12.0					

Table A.II.20 Deaths for all ages and for ages 65 and over by color and sex for aneurysm of aorta and other cardiovascular syphilis: United States, each geographic division and state, 1959-61 (ISC codes 022-023)

Geographic area	All ages					Ages 65 and over				
		White		Nonwhite			White		Nonwhite	
	Total	Male	Female	Male	Female	Total	Male	Female	Male	Female
United States	6,946	3,510	1,231	1,488	717	3,635	2,037	819	543	236
New England	431	288	118	17	8	286	185	90	7	4
Connecticut	94	56	28	6	4	63	40	17	3	3
Maine	23	12	10	1	-	17	8	9	-	-
Massachusetts	234	160	63	9	2	159	105	50	4	-
New Hampshire	33	23	10	-	-	16	9	7	-	-
Rhode Island	32	23	6	1	2	21	14	6	-	1
Vermont	15	14	1	-	-	10	9	1	-	-
Middle Atlantic	1,252	689	237	204	122	679	411	151	70	47
New Jersey	211	126	32	32	21	114	73	23	9	9
New York	509	277	96	87	49	275	172	63	26	14
Pennsylvania	532	286	109	85	52	290	166	65	35	24
East North Central	1,078	577	211	190	100	567	321	137	76	33
Illinois	211	105	42	47	17	107	59	25	19	4
Indiana	145	89	37	11	8	89	52	28	6	3
Michigan	195	101	32	47	15	94	54	19	16	5
Ohio	439	214	85	82	58	228	120	53	34	21
Wisconsin	88	68	15	3	2	49	36	12	1	-
West North Central	552	330	134	69	19	325	187	92	36	10
Iowa	75	43	30	2	-	50	26	23	1	-
Kansas	94	59	18	11	6	53	34	11	4	4
Minnesota	107	82	23	1	1	64	45	17	1	1
Missouri	218	108	49	49	12	118	57	31	25	5
Nebraska	25	14	5	6	-	15	7	3	5	-
North Dakota	8	6	2	-	-	6	4	2	-	-
South Dakota	25	18	7	-	-	19	14	5	-	-

	1,167	389	152	422	204	486	210	100	125	51
South Atlantic										
Delaware	16	10	3	1	2	4	4	-	-	-
District of Columbia	46	6	7	22	11	22	1	7	9	5
Florida	257	87	40	86	44	115	61	30	17	7
Georgia	169	43	10	76	40	58	24	3	25	6
Maryland	216	74	22	79	41	87	31	14	28	14
North Carolina	128	48	17	44	19	53	23	11	15	4
South Carolina	115	36	16	45	18	42	20	10	8	4
Virginia	145	46	19	55	25	64	26	13	14	11
West Virginia	75	39	18	14	4	41	20	12	9	-
East South Central	428	137	37	172	82	174	56	21	67	30
Alabama	150	35	9	65	41	61	12	6	27	16
Kentucky	102	59	17	20	6	43	21	9	11	2
Mississippi	96	16	4	53	23	39	10	1	19	9
Tennessee	80	27	7	34	12	31	13	5	10	3
West South Central	895	365	104	293	133	439	215	73	111	40
Arkansas	85	35	7	31	12	48	24	5	16	3
Louisiana	262	42	19	132	69	112	27	14	48	23
Oklahoma	92	62	13	9	8	54	39	9	3	3
Texas	456	226	65	121	44	225	125	45	44	11
Mountain	237	150	59	21	7	153	98	39	11	5
Arizona	42	23	8	9	2	24	14	6	3	1
Colorado	73	39	25	7	2	48	25	17	4	2
Idaho	23	18	5	-	-	19	15	4	-	-
Montana	28	22	6	-	-	21	17	4	-	-
Nevada	17	12	3	2	-	10	8	1	1	-
New Mexico	24	14	6	1	3	13	6	4	1	2
Utah	16	12	2	2	-	8	6	4	2	-
Wyoming	14	10	4	-	-	10	7	3	-	-
Pacific	906	585	179	100	42	526	354	116	40	16
Alaska	2	-	-	1	1	-	-	-	-	-
California	692	445	133	84	30	393	267	83	32	11
Hawaii	12	1	2	5	4	5	-	-	3	2
Oregon	56	35	11	7	3	29	16	9	3	1
Washington	144	104	33	3	4	99	71	24	2	2

Table A.II.21 Age-adjusted death rates per 100,000 population for all ages and for ages 65 and over, by color and sex for aneurysm of aorta and other cardiovascular syphilis: United States, each geographic division and state, 1959-61 (ISC codes 022-023)

Geographic area	All ages					Ages 65 and over				
		White		Nonwhite			White		Nonwhite	
	Total	Male	Female	Male	Female	Total	Male	Female	Male	Female
United States	1.1	1.3	0.4	5.8	2.6	7.3	9.8	3.1	30.4	12.0
New England	1.0	1.5	0.5	5.7*	2.6*	8.4	13.0	4.5	34.0*	18.2*
Connecticut	1.0*	1.3	0.5	5.8*	3.7*	8.6	12.7	4.1*	51.2*	42.0*
Maine	0.5*	0.7*	0.4*	24.9*	-	5.0*	5.5*	4.6*	-	-
Massachusetts	1.1	1.7	0.5*	5.7*	1.3*	9.1	14.8	4.8	34.7*	-
New Hampshire	1.4*	2.1*	0.7*	-	-	8.0*	10.4*	5.9*	-	-
Rhode Island	0.9*	1.5*	0.3*	4.6*	9.1*	8.0*	12.5*	4.0*	-	59.5*
Vermont	0.9*	2.0*	0.0*	-	-	7.5*	16.0*	.7*	-	-
Middle Atlantic	0.9	1.2	0.3	5.8	3.1	6.7	9.6	2.7	34.5	19.6
New Jersey	1.0	1.3	0.3*	5.2*	3.1*	6.8	10.4	2.5*	24.2*	20.6*
New York	0.8	0.9	0.3	5.1	2.4*	5.4	7.9	2.3	29.1*	12.2*
Pennsylvania	1.2	1.5	0.5	7.2	4.2	8.5	11.5	3.5	46.9*	29.5*
East North Central	0.8	1.0	0.3	5.4	2.7	5.6	7.4	2.5	34.7	14.0*
Illinois	0.6	0.6	0.2*	3.7*	1.2*	3.7	4.8	1.6*	24.6*	4.7*
Indiana	0.9	1.2	0.4*	3.1*	2.2*	6.5	8.9	3.8*	24.0*	12.3*
Michigan	0.8	0.9	0.3*	5.5*	1.8*	4.9	6.3	1.9*	34.0*	9.8*
Ohio	1.3	1.4	0.5	8.1	5.6	8.4	10.4	3.6	52.2*	30.4*
Wisconsin	0.6	0.9	0.2*	3.7	2.4*	4.0*	6.4*	1.7*	21.1*	-
West North Central	0.9	1.2	0.4	7.5	2.0*	6.4	8.2	3.2	51.7*	13.6*
Iowa	0.6	0.8*	0.4*	4.6*	-	5.0*	5.9*	4.0*	31.0*	-
Kansas	1.1	1.6	0.4*	7.7*	3.6*	7.2	10.9*	2.4*	32.1*	30.6*
Minnesota	0.8	1.3	0.3*	1.8*	2.1*	6.0	8.9*	3.0*	26.9*	30.4*
Missouri	1.3	1.4	0.5*	8.4*	1.9*	8.1	9.3	3.8*	56.7*	10.5*
Nebraska	0.4*	0.5*	0.2*	12.4*	-	3.2*	3.1*	1.2*	146.6*	-
North Dakota	0.4*	0.6*	0.2*	-	-	3.6*	4.9*	2.3*	-	-
South Dakota	0.9*	1.3*	0.6*	-	-	8.6*	13.3*	4.2*	-	-

South Atlantic	1.4	1.2	0.4	6.2	2.7	7.7	8.8	3.3	26.2	9.1*
Delaware	1.2*	1.7*	0.6*	1.2*	2.6*	3.6*	9.4*	-	-	-
District of Columbia	1.6*	0.9*	0.5*	4.8	2.1*	10.4*	1.3*	7.8*	33.7*	14.1*
Florida	1.4	1.0	0.4*	8.2	4.1*	6.9	8.2	3.8*	25.7*	9.9*
Georgia	1.5	1.1*	0.2*	6.0	2.6*	6.7	8.3*	0.7*	26.1*	4.7*
Maryland	2.3	2.0	0.5*	12.4	6.5*	12.9	12.3*	3.9*	70.1*	33.8*
North Carolina	1.0	1.0*	0.3*	3.5*	1.4*	5.7*	6.9*	2.7*	17.4*	4.0*
South Carolina	1.9	1.9*	0.6*	5.5*	1.8*	9.3*	15.4*	5.1*	12.7*	4.9*
Virginia	1.2	1.0*	0.3*	5.3	2.2*	7.3	8.5*	3.1*	18.1*	12.7*
West Virginia	1.1	1.3*	0.5*	7.3*	2.7*	7.7*	8.1*	4.7*	63.3*	-
East South Central	1.1	0.9	0.2*	4.7	2.1	5.6	5.0	1.4*	22.0	8.8*
Alabama	1.5	1.0*	0.2*	5.2	2.9*	7.9	4.9*	1.7*	26.8*	13.2*
Kentucky	1.0	1.3	0.3*	5.2*	1.7*	5.0*	5.7*	2.0*	35.3*	5.8*
Mississippi	1.4	0.7*	0.2*	4.4*	1.8*	6.9*	6.2*	0.4*	17.4*	8.2*
Tennessee	0.7	0.6*	0.1*	4.1*	1.4*	3.5*	3.8*	1.2*	15.6*	4.1*
West South Central	1.6	1.6	0.4	7.6	3.2	10.3	13.0	3.7	35.3	11.5*
Arkansas	1.2	1.2*	0.2*	5.0*	1.8*	8.4*	10.8*	2.0*	28.4*	5.3*
Louisiana	2.7	1.3*	0.5*	10.3	4.7	15.5	12.4*	5.2*	45.7*	18.6*
Oklahoma	1.0	1.5	0.3*	2.8*	2.3*	7.1	12.4*	2.0*	10.6*	10.8*
Texas	1.5	1.8	0.4	7.4	2.6*	10.0	13.9	4.1*	35.3*	8.2*
Mountain	1.1	1.5	0.6	5.3*	2.3*	9.7	13.2	4.8*	42.6*	24.1*
Arizona	1.1*	1.3*	0.4*	6.2*	1.8*	8.9*	11.2*	4.7*	29.3*	13.0*
Colorado	1.2	1.4*	0.8*	11.7*	3.2*	10.0*	11.9*	6.0*	88.8*	46.1*
Idaho	1.0*	1.5*	0.4*	-	-	11.1*	17.6*	4.6*	-	-
Montana	1.1*	1.7*	0.5*	-	-	10.8*	17.1*	4.4*	-	-
Nevada	2.1*	2.8*	0.9*	9.2*	5.8*	18.4*	28.6*	5.7*	75.8*	58.3*
New Mexico	1.1*	1.4*	0.6*	1.6*	-	8.7*	8.5*	-	23.1*	-
Utah	0.7*	1.1*	0.2*	7.8*	-	4.5*	7.4*	-	113.4*	-
Wyoming	1.3*	1.8*	0.8*	-	-	12.2*	17.0*	7.7*	-	-
Pacific	1.2	1.8	0.5	4.3	2.2*	9.3	14.8	3.7	28.5*	13.5*
Alaska	0.4*	-	-	2.0*	2.6*	9.5	15.4	3.5	-	-
California	1.3	1.9	0.5	5.6	2.2*	5.9*	-	-	36.1*	13.7*
Hawaii	0.9*	0.6*	1.1*	0.9*	1.0*	5.1*	6.2*	2.9*	8.2*	7.4*
Oregon	0.8*	1.1*	0.3*	13.3*	7.7*	-	-	5.1*	76.8*	45.0*
Washington	1.3	2.0	0.6*	2.6*	4.6*	11.9	18.5	-	26.2*	34.2*

Table A.II.22 Age-adjusted death rates per 100,000 population for aneurysm of aorta and other cardiovascular syphilis by color and sex, for all ages for metropolitan and non-metropolitan counties in each geographic division United States, 1959-61 (ISC codes 022-023)

Sex; geographic division	White Metropolitan counties			White Non-metropolitan counties	Nonwhite Metropolitan counties		Nonwhite Non-metropolitan counties
	Total	with central city	without central city		Total	without central city	
Male							
United States	1.4	1.4	1.2*	1.1	6.8	5.9	4.3*
New England	1.6*	1.6*	1.5*	1.4*	5.2*	0.0*	12.6*
Middle Atlantic	1.2	1.2*	1.1*	1.2*	5.9*	5.8	4.7*
East North Central	1.0*	1.0*	1.0*	1.0*	5.6*	2.2*	3.0*
West North Central	1.8*	1.9*	1.2*	.8*	8.0*	8.8*	6.3*
South Atlantic	1.4*	1.4*	1.2*	1.0*	7.9*	6.8	4.6*
East South Central	1.4*	1.3*	2.0*	.7*	6.3*	6.4*	3.7*
West South Central	1.9*	2.0*	1.1*	1.4*	11.0*	6.5*	5.0*
Mountain	1.5*	1.6*	1.0*	1.5*	8.8*	0.0*	3.5*
Pacific	1.8*	1.7*	2.0*	1.9*	4.8*	7.3*	2.5*
Female							
United States	.4	.4*	.3*	.3*	3.0*	4.1	2.0*
New England	.5*	.5*	.7*	.4*	2.9*	0.0*	0.0*
Middle Atlantic	.3*	.4*	.3*	.4*	3.1*	2.4*	2.4*
East North Central	.3*	.3*	.3*	.3*	2.7*	4.1*	2.7*
West North Central	.5*	.6*	.2*	.3*	2.2*	3.6*	1.2*
South Atlantic	.4*	.4*	.3*	.4*	3.8*	6.0	1.7*
East South Central	.3*	.3*	.6*	.2*	2.3*	2.4*	1.8*
West South Central	.4*	.4*	.7*	.4*	4.0*	5.9*	2.5*
Mountain	.5*	.5*	.5*	.6*	1.5*	0.0*	3.1*
Pacific	.4*	.4*	.6*	.5*	2.0*	6.5*	3.3*

Table A.II.23 Death rates per 100,000 population for aneurysm of aorta and other cardiovascular syphilis by marital status, color, and sex; United States age-adjusted for ages 15 and over, 15-64, and 65 and over; geographic divisions for ages 15-64 only, 1959-61 (ISC codes 022-023)

Sex, age, area	White				Nonwhite			
	Single	Married	Widowed	Divorced	Single	Married	Widowed	Divorced
Male								
United States								
15 and over	2.1*	1.5	2.3*	4.1*	10.4*	6.4	12.3*	16.4*
15-64	1.1*	0.8	1.3*	2.7*	7.1*	4.5	10.1*	10.3*
65 and over	12.6	9.0	12.2	18.2*	42.9*	25.8	34.1	76.7*
15-64								
New England	1.2*	0.8*	1.1*	1.4*	6.6*	4.0*	5.5*	11.6*
Middle Atlantic	0.9*	0.7*	0.7*	2.5*	5.5*	3.9*	12.9*	7.5*
East North Central	0.8*	0.6*	0.7*	3.1*	3.6*	4.0*	5.2*	7.4*
West North Central	1.4*	0.7*	1.3*	4.4*	8.9*	4.4*	10.8*	9.9*
South Atlantic	1.3*	0.8*	1.9*	1.6*	10.5*	5.2*	11.4*	12.3*
East South Central	0.8*	0.8*	1.2*	1.7*	8.1*	4.1*	5.8*	8.0*
West South Central	0.9*	1.0*	1.9*	2.9*	11.9*	5.8*	18.0*	18.1*
Mountain	0.2*	0.8*	3.6*	1.1*	13.2*	2.8*	4.6*	10.5*
Pacific	1.4*	0.9*	2.7*	3.2*	2.9*	2.8*	3.5*	9.2*
Females								
United States								
15 and over	0.4*	0.4	0.7*	0.9*	5.1*	2.4	4.7*	5.0*
15-64	0.3*	0.2*	0.4*	0.5*	4.0*	1.7	3.9*	3.6*
65 and over	2.0*	2.9	3.5	5.7*	15.8*	9.3*	12.3	18.9*
15-64								
New England	0.3*	0.2*	0.1*	0.2*	-	1.5*	3.6*	-
Middle Atlantic	0.2*	0.2*	0.2*	0.4*	3.8*	1.7*	2.8*	3.9*
East North Central	0.3*	0.2*	0.3*	0.4*	3.3*	2.2*	2.8*	3.0*
West North Central	0.7*	0.2*	0.5*	0.3*	-	0.7*	3.2*	2.1*
South Atlantic	-	0.2*	0.4*	0.5*	5.2*	1.9*	4.5*	2.5*
East South Central	-	0.1*	0.2*	0.6*	2.5*	1.3*	3.1*	3.3*
West South Central	0.2*	0.2*	0.2*	0.7*	7.3*	1.9*	6.7*	6.1*
Mountain	-	0.3*	0.2*	0.7*	-	0.7*	1.8*	-
Pacific	0.2*	0.3*	1.0*	0.4*	1.1*	1.4*	2.9*	4.2*

Table A.II.24   Age-adjusted death rates per 100,000 population for aneurysm of aorta and other cardiovascular syphilis for the white native-born and white foreign-born by sex, for all ages, under 65 years, and 65 and over in each geographic division: United States, 1959-61 (ISC codes 022-023)

Nativity; sex; age	New England	Middle Atlantic	East North Central	West North Central	South Atlantic	East South Central	West South Central	Mountain	Pacific
White native born									
Male									
All ages	1.6*	1.2*	1.0*	1.1*	1.2*	0.9*	1.5*	1.4*	1.8*
Under 65	0.8*	0.5*	0.5*	0.6*	0.6*	0.6*	0.7*	0.6*	0.8*
65 and over	12.5	10.8	7.7	7.9*	8.7	5.2*	12.9	11.9*	15.0
Female									
All ages	0.5*	0.4*	0.3*	0.4*	0.4*	0.2*	0.4*	0.5*	0.4*
Under 65	0.2*	0.2*	0.1*	0.2*	0.2*	0.1*	0.1*	0.2*	0.2*
65 and over	5.1	3.1	2.5	3.2	3.3	1.5*	3.8	4.3*	3.5
White foreign born									
Male									
All ages	1.3*	1.1*	0.8*	2.2*	1.5*	3.1*	4.3*	2.3*	1.9*
Under 65	0.4*	0.6*	0.4*	1.5*	0.8*	2.9*	3.4*	0.8*	0.9*
65 and over	13.6	8.1	6.6	11.1*	11.4*	5.9*	17.1*	22.6*	15.1
Female									
All ages	0.6*	0.3*	0.4*	0.5*	0.5*	0.5*	1.1*	0.7*	0.5*
Under 65	0.4*	0.2*	0.2*	0.3*	0.2*	0.0*	1.0*	0.2*	0.2*
65 and over	3.5*	2.0*	2.5*	3.2*	4.4*	7.1*	2.3*	7.8*	4.7*

Table A.II.25   First admissions to mental institutions[a] for all psychoses and for psychoses due to syphilis: United States, 1922, 1933-47, 1960, and 1965

Year	Number of first admissions					Rates per 100,000 population			
	All psychoses	General paresis (syphilis)	Other syphilis of the central nervous system	Total psychoses due to syphilis	Percent of all psychoses due to syphilis	All psychoses	General paresis (syphilis)	Other syphilis of the central nervous system	Total psychoses due to syphilis
1922	64,689	6,260	892	7,152	11.1	58.8	5.7	0.8	6.5
1933	80,974	6,889	1,429	8,318	10.3	64.5	5.5	1.1	6.6
1934	80,575	6,869	1,428	8,297	10.3	63.8	5.4	1.1	6.6
1935	83,943	6,974	1,432	8,406	10.0	66.0	5.5	1.1	6.6
1936	88,259	7,070	1,343	8,413	9.5	68.9	5.5	1.0	6.6
1937	89,858	6,918	1,357	8,275	9.2	69.8	5.4	1.1	6.4
1938	89,461	6,962	1,255	8,217	9.2	68.9	5.4	1.0	6.3
1939	90,143	7,261	1,364	8,625	9.6	68.9	5.5	1.0	6.6
1940	87,592	6,558	1,136	7,694	8.8	66.5	5.0	0.9	5.8
1941	94,176	6,938	1,145	8,083	8.6	70.8	5.2	0.9	6.1
1942	94,310	6,786	1,139	7,925	8.4	70.5	5.1	0.9	5.9
1943	92,126	6,316	968	7,284	7.9	68.8	4.7	0.7	5.4
1944	93,821	6,179	889	7,068	7.5	70.8	4.7	0.7	5.3
1945	95,119	6,008	889	6,897	7.3	72.0	4.6	0.7	5.2
1946	101,444	5,746	801	6,547	6.5	72.5	4.1	0.6	4.7
1947	100,938	5,349	743	6,102	6.0	70.4	3.7	0.5	4.3
1960	122,000[b]	563	179	742	0.6	64.0	0.3	0.1	0.4
1965	---	167	65	232	---	---	0.1	0.0	0.1

Source: The National Institute of Mental Health, Patients in Mental Institutions (annual publications) and Communicable Disease Center, Venereal Disease Branch, The Journal of Venereal Disease Information, November 1949.

[a] Excluding admissions to Veterans Administration hospitals.

[b] Classification procedures change and estimates were made for comparative purposes with previous years data.

Table A.II.26   Median age of reported syphilis deaths: United States,
selected years from 1933 to 1965

Year	Syphilis and its sequelae					General paralysis All cases	Tabes dorsalis All cases	Aneurysm of aorta All cases	All other cases
	All Cases	White		Nonwhite					
		Male	Female	Male	Female				
1933	48.2	52.8	49.0	43.2	36.5	48.6	60.6	57.4	44.1
1939	50.5	55.7	51.5	45.0	37.5	50.5	62.4	56.4	46.1
1940	51.5	55.9	51.8	46.0	39.1	51.1	62.6	55.8	47.5
1960	65.2	66.7	68.4	61.2	59.0	61.8	67.7	66.8	63.8
1965	68.1	69.4	71.0	63.0	62.4	63.7	72.3	69.5	65.5

Note: The median age of death for all causes was 58.2 in 1933 and 69.9 in
1965. The median age of death for all other cardiovascular syphilis, included with
Other in above table, was 58.7 in 1950, 64.1 in 1960, and 66.4 in 1965.

Table A.II.27   Deaths and death rates per 100,000 population
for syphilis and its sequelae: selected countries,
1960 and 1965 (ISC, Seventh Revision, 1955
Abbreviated List, B-3)

Country	Deaths		Death rate	
	1965	1960	1965	1960
Africa				
Mauritius	1	4	0.1	0.6
South Africa:				
White population	7b	54	0.2	1.8
Asiatic population	1b	5	0.2	1.1
Colored population	47b	110	2.9	7.3
UAR (Egypt)	30c	62	0.2	0.5
America				
Canada	105	172	0.5	1.0
Chile[a]	106d	173	1.3	2.2
Colombia	226	234	1.3	1.5
Costa Rica	19	12	1.3	1.0
Dominican Republic[a]	72c	99	g	3.3
El Salvador	22c	81	g	g
Guatemala	3d,e	5e	0.1	0.1
Mexico	310	678	0.7	1.9
Panama	17	7	1.4	0.7
Puerto Rico	40	43	1.5	1.8
Trinidad & Tobago	40d	43	4.2	5.1
United States	2,434	2,945	1.3	1.6
Venezuela[a]	141	196	g	g
Asia				
China: Taiwan	31e	152	0.2	1.4
Hong Kong	53	61	1.4	2.0
Israel	5	12	0.2	0.6
Japan	1,581f	2,068	1.6	2.2
Philippines	40d	191f	0.1	0.7
Singapore[a]	19	34	1.0	2.1
Thailand	11d	38	g	g

A.II.27 cont.

Country	Deaths		Death rate	
	1965	1960	1965	1960
Europe				
Austria	87	131	1.2	1.9
Belgium	90[c]	146	1.0	1.6
Bulgaria	25	43	0.3	0.5
Czechoslovakia	258[d]	356	1.8	2.6
Denmark	41[d]	59	0.9	1.3
Finland	69	92	1.5	2.1
France	862[e]	933[c]	1.8	2.0
Germany:				
Federal Republic	532[d]	600	0.9	1.1
West Berlin	81[d]	91	3.7	4.1
Greece	31	28	0.4	0.3
Hungary	140	185	1.4	1.9
Ireland	5	6	0.2	0.2
Italy	689[d]	1,024	1.3	2.1
Malta[a]	2	5	0.6	1.5
Netherlands	117	162	1.0	1.4
Norway	46[d]	60	1.2	1.7
Poland	239	148	0.8	0.5
Portugal[a]	177	241	1.9	2.7
Spain[a]	760[c,e]	940[e]	2.4	3.1
Sweden	24	36	0.3	0.5
Switzerland	56[d]	80	1.0	1.5
United Kingdom:				
England and Wales	856	944	1.8	2.1
Northern Ireland	16	29	1.1	2.0
Scotland	52	64	1.0	1.2
Yugoslavia	212[d]	368	g	g
Oceania				
Australia[a]	77	76	0.7	0.7
New Zealand	10	14	0.4	0.6

Source: United Nations, Demographic Yearbook, 1966,
New York, 1967. Table 20, p. 484 ff.

aDeaths coded according to the categories of
the Sixth (1948) Revision of the ISC.
bData relate to 1962.
cData relate to 1963.
dData relate to 1964.
eExcludes children born alive, but dead before
registration of their birth.
fEstimated or provisional.
gRates not computed either because deaths due
to senility, ill-defined and unknown causes
(B-45) exceed 25 percent of total deaths, or
because deaths from all causes number less than 1,000.

Notes

Chapter 1. The History of Syphilis
   1. R. R. Willcox, "Venereal Disease in the Bible," *British Journal of Venereal Diseases,* 25:28–33 (1949).
   2. R. C. Holcomb, "Christopher Columbus, and the American Origin of Syphilis," *United States Naval Medical Bulletin,* 32:423 (1934).
   3. William L. Fleming, "Syphilis Through the Ages," *The Medical Clinics of North America,* 48: 587–612 (1964).
   4. William A. Pusey, *The History and Epidemiology of Syphilis* (Springfield, 1933).
   5. L. W. Harrison, "The Origin of Syphilis," *The British Journal of Venereal Diseases,* 35: 1–7 (1959).
   6. Herbert U. Williams, "The Origin and Antiquity of Syphilis: The Evidence of Diseased Bones," *Archives of Pathology,* 13: 976 (June 1932).
   7. Thomas A. Cockburn, *The Evolution and Eradication of Infectious Diseases* (Baltimore, 1963).
   8. Ellis H. Hudson, "Treponematosis and African Slavery," *British Journal of Venereal Diseases,* 40: 43–52 (March 1964).
   9. Ellis H. Hudson, "Treponematosis and Anthropology," *Annals of Internal Medicine,* 58: 1037–48 (June 1963).
   10. Ellis H. Hudson, "Treponematosis and Pilgrimage," *The American Journal of the Medical Sciences,* 246: 645–656 (December 1963).
   11. Cockburn, *The Evolution and Eradication of Infectious Diseases.*
   12. Hudson, "Treponematosis and African Slavery," pp. 43–52.
   13. Hudson, "Treponematosis and Anthropology," pp. 1037–48.
   14. Hudson, "Treponematosis and Pilgrimage," pp. 645–656.

Chapter 2. Evolution of Treatment
   1. J. Johnston Abraham, "Some Account of the History of the Treatment of Syphilis," *British Journal of Venereal Diseases,* 24:156 (1948).
   2. John H. Stokes, Herman Beerman, and Norman R. Ingraham, *Modern Clinical Syphilology,* 3rd ed. (Philadelphia, 1944), p. 216.
   3. Abraham, "Some Account of the History of the Treatment of Syphilis." p. 154.
   4. John H. Stokes, *Modern Clinical Syphilology,* 2nd ed. (Philadelphia, 1934), p. 766.
   5. *Ibid.,* p. 754.
   6. Thomas Parran as cited by Odin W. Anderson, *Syphilis and Society,* (Chicago, 1965), p. 20.
   7. Stokes, *Modern Clinical Syphilology,* 2nd ed., p. 1178.
   8. J. F. Mahoney, R. D. Arnold, and A. Harris. "Penicillin Treatment of Early Syphilis: A Preliminary Report," *Journal of Venereal Disease Information,* 24:355–357 (December 1943).

Chapter 3. The Diagnosis and Treatment of Syphilis

1. Edvin Bruusgaard, "Uber das Schicksal der nicht spezifisch behandelten Luetiker," Archiv fur Dermatologie und Syphilis, 157:309 (1929) as cited in *Journal of Chronic Diseases*, 2:311–344 (September 1955). (See footnote number 3).

2. Trygve Gjestland, "The Oslo Study of Untreated Syphilis: An Epidemiologic Investigation of the Natural Course of Untreated Syphilis Based on a Restudy of the Boeck-Bruusgaard Material," *Acta Dermato-Venereologica*, vol. 35, supplementum 34 (Oslo, 1955).

3. E. Gurney Clark and Niels Danbolt, "The Oslo Study of the Natural History of Untreated Syphilis," *Journal of Chronic Diseases*, 2:311–344 (September 1955).

4. Donald H. Rockwell, Anne R. Yobs, and M. Brittain Moore, "The Tuskegee Study of Untreated Syphilis," *Archives of Internal Medicine*, 114:792–798 (December 1964).

5. Seward E. Miller, *A Textbook of Clinical Pathology* (Baltimore, 1955), p. 997.

6. Herman Beerman, "The Problem of Reinoculation of Human Beings with *Spirochaeta Pallida*," *American Journal of Syphilis, Gonorrhea, and Venereal Diseases*, 30:173 (March 1946).

7. Ira L. Schamberg and Howard P. Steiger, "Syphilitic Relapse vs. Reinfection," *The Journal of Venereal Disease Information*, 29:94 (April 1948).

8. Harold J. Magnuson, Evan W. Thomas, Sidney Olansky, Bernard I. Kaplan, Lopo de Mello, and John C. Cutler, "Inoculation Syphilis in Human Volunteers," *Medicine*, 35:33–82 (February 1956).

9. John H. Stokes, *Modern Clinical Syphilology*, 2nd ed. (Philadelphia, 1934) p. 1239.

10. John H. Stokes, Herman Beerman, and Norman R. Ingraham, *Modern Clinical Syphilology*, 3rd ed. (Philadelphia, 1944) p. 1077.

11. J. Earle Moore and Charles F. Mohr, "Biologically False Positive Serologic Tests for Syphilis," *The Journal of the American Medical Association*, 150:468 (October 1952).

12. Harry Eagle, "On the Specificity of Serologic Tests for Syphilis as Determined by 40,545 Tests in a College Student Population," *American Journal of Syphilis, Gonorrhea, and Venereal Diseases*, 25:14 (1941).

13. John A. Kolmer and Elsa R. Lynch, "False Positive Reactions in the Serologic Diagnosis of Syphilis," *American Journal of Clinical Pathology*, 23:855 (September 1953).

Chapter 4. Venereal Disease Casefinding and Control Measures in the Twentieth Century

1. Joseph F. Siler, *The Prevention and Control of Venereal Diseases in the Army of the United States of America*, Army Medical Bulletin No. 67 (Carlisle Barracks, Pa., 1943), p. 100.

2. Thomas Parran, *Shadow On The Land* (New York: Reynal and Hitchcock, 1937).

3. J. F. Mahoney et al., "Experimental Gonococcic Urethritis in Human Volunteers," *American Journal of Syphilis, Gonorrhea, and the Venereal Diseases,* 30:1 (January 1946).

4. James D. Thayer and M. B. Moore, Jr., "Gonorrhea — Present Knowledge, Research, and Control Efforts," *The Medical Clinics of North America,* 48:762 (May 1964).

5. John W. Morse and A. P. Iskrant, "Syphilis Casefinding Through Education," *Journal of Venereal Disease Information,* 32:150 (June 1951).

6. *Syphilis Epidemiology, Report 2* (Atlanta, Ga., July 23, 1965), p. 14.

7. S. W. Trythall, "The Premarital Law: History and Survey in Michigan," *Journal of the American Medical Association,* 187:900 (June 8, 1964).

8. *Today's VD Control Problem: Joint Statement,* The American Public Health Association, The American Social Health Association, The American Venereal Disease Association, The Association of State and Territorial Health Officers with the cooperation of the American Medical Association (New York, January 1967), pp. 13–14.

9. William J. Brown and E. J. Sunkes, "A Recent Study of Results of Premarital Serologic Testing in a Southern State," *Southern Medical Journal,* 52:709 (June 1959).

10. P. K. Condit and A. Frank Brewer, "Premarital Examination Laws—Are They Worthwhile? California Experience with 2,000,000 Examinations," *American Journal of Public Health,* 48:880 (July 1953).

11. Trythall, "Premarital Law in Michigan," p. 900.

12. *Today's VD Control Problem: Joint Statement,* p. 13.

13. William J. Brown and J. A. Mahoney, "Serologic Tests for Syphilis: A Profile of Hospital Practice," *Journal of the American Hospital Association,* 37:65–69 (Nov. 1, 1963).

14. "New Edition of Hospital Accreditation Standards," *Journal of the American Medical Association,* 161:242 (May 19, 1956).

15. *Today's VD Control Problem: Joint Statement,* p. 7.

16. Brown and Mahoney, "Serologic Tests for Syphilis," p. 66.

17. *Findings on the Serologic Test for Syphilis in Adults,* PHS Publication No. 1000, Series 11, No. 9 (Washington, D.C., 1965), p. 4.

18. John H. Stokes et al., "Syphilis in Industry: A Review of Problems and Policy," *American Journal of the Medical Sciences,* 196:600 (October 1938).

19. Otis L. Anderson, "The Control of Venereal Diseases Among Industrial Workers," *American Journal of Syphilis, Gonorrhea, and Venereal Diseases,* 27:432 (July 1943).

20. Ross Taggart et al., "District of Columbia Blood Testing Survey for Syphilis in Selected Industries and Trades," *Medical Annals of the District of Columbia,* 25:73 (February 1956).

21. *The Eradication of Syphilis.* A Task Force Report to the Surgeon General, Public Health Service, on Syphilis Control in the United States, PHS Publication No. 918 (Washington D.C., 1962).

22. M. B. Moore, Jr., et al., "Epidemiologic Treatment of Contacts to Infectious Syphilis," *Public Health Reports,* 78:966 (November 1963).

Chapter 5. Morbidity

1. Joseph Siler, "The Prevention and Control of Venereal Diseases in the Army of the United States of America," *Army Medical Bulletin No. 67,* (Pennsylvania, 1943), p. 100.

2. *Findings on the Serologic Test for Syphilis in Adults,* PHS Publication No. 1000, Series 11, No. 9 (Washington, D. C., 1965).

3. *Today's VD Control Problem: Joint Statement* (New York, March 1964), pp. 74-75.

4. John W. Lentz and Herman Beerman, "The Treatment of Venereal Diseases in Private Practice in Philadelphia," *American Journal of Syphilis, Gonorrhea, and Venereal Diseases,* 37: 427-438 (September 1953).

5. Arthur Curtis, "National Survey of Venereal Disease Treatment," *Journal of the American Medical Association,* 86: 46-49 (October 1963).

6. Odin W. Anderson, *Syphilis and Society: Problems of Control in the United States, 1912-1964,* (Chicago: University of Chicago, 1965).

7. *Venereal Disease Branch Report, Fiscal Year 1966,* Public Health Service (Atlanta, Georgia).

8. *Venereal Disease in Canada, Annual Report, 1964,* Epidemiology Division, Department of National Health and Welfare (Ottawa).

9. *Findings on the Serologic Test for Syphilis in Adults,* PHS Publication No. 1000, Series 11, No. 9 (Washington, D. C., 1965).

10. Ibid.

Chapter 6. Gonorrhea

1. *Venereal Disease Branch Report, Fiscal Year 1966,* Communicable Disease Center, Public Health Service, U. S. Department of Health, Education and Welfare (Atlanta, Georgia, 1966).

2. A. C. Curtis, "National Survey of Venereal Disease Treatment," *Journal of the American Medical Association,* 186:46-49 (Oct. 5, 1963).

3. "Control of Gonococcal Infections," *World Health Organization Chronical,* 18:14-15 (January 1964).

4. H. Pariser, A. D. Farmer, and A. F. Marino, "Asymptomatic Gonorrhea in the Male," *Southern Medical Journal,* 57:680-690 (June 1964).

5. Medical News Section, *Journal of the American Medical Association,* 193:23-24 (Aug. 23, 1965).

6. *The Gonococcus,* PHS Publication No. 499 (Washington, D. C.: U. S. Government Printing Office (1962) p. 4.

7. W. E. Deacon, "Fluorescent Antibody Methods for *Neisseria Gonorrhoeae* Identification," *World Health Organization Bulletin,* 24:349-355 (1961).

8. D. S. Kellogg, Jr., and W. E. Deacon, "A New Rapid Immuno-fluorescent Staining Technique for Identification of *Treponema pallidum* and *Neisseria Gonorrhoeae*," *Proceedings of the Society for Experimental Biology and Medicine*, 115:963-965 (1964).

9. W. L. Peacock, Jr., and J. D. Thayer, "Direct Fluorescent Antibody Technique Using Flazo Orange Counterstain in Identification of *Neisseria Gonorrhoeae*," *Public Health Reports*, 79:1119-22 (December 1964).

10. L. A. White and D. S. Kellogg, Jr., "*Neisseria Gonorrhoeae* Identification in Direct Smears by a Fluorescent Antibody-Counterstain Method," *Applied Microbiology*, 13:171-174 (March 1965).

11. James D. Thayer and J. E. Martin, Jr., "A Selective Medium for the Cultivation of *Neisseria Gonorrhoeae* and *Neisseria Meningitidis*," *Public Health Reports*, 79:49-57 (January 1964).

12. James D. Thayer and J. E. Martin, Jr., "Improved Medium Selective for Cultivation of *Neisseria Gonorrhoeae* and *Neisseria Meningitidis*," *Public Health Reports*, 81:559-562 (June 1966).

13. P. C. Miller, "Experimental Gonococcal Infection," *Gonococcus and Gonococcal Infection*, The American Association for the Advancement of Science, Publication No. 11 (Lancaster, Pa.: The Science Press, 1939) p. 20-22.

14. P. C. Miller, M. J. Drell, V. Moeller, and M. Bohnhoff, "Experimental Gonococcal Infection of the Rabbit's Eye," *Journal of Infectious Diseases*, 77:193-200 (1945).

15. A. B. Ackerman and R. Calabria, "Asymptomatic Gonorrhea and the Gonococcal Carrier State, and Gonococcemia in Men," *The Journal of the American Medical Association*, 196:101-103 (Apr. 4, 1966).

16. P. F. Sparling, A. R. Yobs, T. E. Billings, and J. F. Hackney, "Spectinomycin Sulfate and Aqueous Procaine Penicillin G. in Treatment of Female Gonorrhea Antimicrobial Agents and Chemotherapy - 1965," *Antimicrobial Agents and Chemotherapy* (American Society for Microbiology, 1965), 5:689-692.

17. A. E. Wilkinson, "A Note on the Use of Thayer and Martin's Selective Medium for *Neisseria Gonorrhoeae*," *British Journal of Venereal Diseases*, 41:60-61 (March 1965).

18. J. E. Martin, W. L. Peacock, and J. D. Thayer, "Further Studies with a Selective Medium for Cultivating *Neisseria Gonorrhoeae*," *British Journal of Venereal Diseases*, 41:199-201 (September 1965).

19. G. Reising and D. S. Kellogg, Jr., "Detection of Gonococcal Antibody," *Proceedings of the Society for Experimental Biology and Medicine*, 120:660-663 (1965).

20. B. Magnusson and J. Kjellander, "Gonococcal Complement-fixation Test in Complicated and Uncomplicated Gonorrhea," *British Journal of Venereal Diseases*, 41:127-131 (June 1965).

21. I. R. Cohen, "Natural and Immune Human Antibodies Reactive with Antigens of Virulent *Neisseria Gonorrhoeae*, Immunoglobulins G, M, and A." In publication.

22. "Gonorrhea, Interim Recommended Treatment Schedules, July 1965," insert in *Notes on Modern Management of V. D.*, PHS Publication No. 859 (Washington, D.C.: U.S. Government Printing Office, 1962).

Chapter 7. Mortality Caused by Syphilis and It's Sequelae and Other Late Manifestations of Untreated Venereal Disease

1. George H. Van Buren, "Some Things You Can't Prove by Mortality Statistics," *Vital Statistics-Special Reports,* vol. 12, no. 13 (1940), pp. 191-210.

2. Halbert L. Dunn and William Shackley, "Comparison of Cause-of-Death Assignments by the 1929 and 1938 Revisions of the International List: Deaths in the United States, 1940," *Vital Statistics-Special Reports,* vol. 19, no. 14 (1944), pp. 153-278.

3. "Comparability Ratios Based on Mortality Statistics for the Fifth and Sixth Revisions: United States, 1950," *Vital Statistics-Special Reports,* vol. 51, no. 3 (1964), pp. 179-246.

4. *Vital Statistics of the United States, 1955,* Vital Statistics Division, National Center for Health Statistics, vol. I, p. xxv.

5. "Comparability Ratios Based on Mortality Statistics for the Fifth and Sixth Revisions: United States 1950."

6. "Comparability of Mortality Statistics for the Sixth and Seventh Revisions: United States, 1958," *Vital Statistics-Special Reports,* vol. 51, no. 4 (1965), p. 278.

7. *Vital Statistics of the United States, 1959,* vol. I, pp. 1-18.

8. Kurt Pohlen, "The Frequency of Syphilis and Its Sequels According to Clinical and Autopsy Finding," *Dermatologische Wochenschrift,* 105:1469 (1937), as cited in *Journal of Venereal Disease Information,* 19:184 (June 1938).

9. *Ibid.*

10. *Vital Statistics of the United States, 1958,* vol. I, pp. 6-29 and vol. II, p. 93.

11. *Vital Statistics of the United States, 1955, Supplement: Mortality Data Multiple Causes of Death.*

12. *Vital Statistics of the United States, 1940,* vol. I, p. 576.

13. *Vital Statistics of the United States, 1955, Supplement: Mortality Data Multiple Causes of Death.*

14. M. Nicoll and M. T. Bellows, "Effect of a Confidential Inquiry on the Recorded Mortality from Syphilis and Alcoholism," *American Journal of Public Health,* 24:813-820 (1934).

15. Kurt Pohlen, "The Frequency of Syphilis and Its Sequels According to Clinical and Autopsy Finding," p. 1469.

16. Trygve Gjestland, "The Oslo Study of Untreated Syphilis: An Epidemiologic Investigation of the Natural Course of Untreated Syphilis Based on a Restudy of the Boeck-Bruusgaard Material," *Acta Dermato-Venereologica,* vol. 35, supplementum 34 (Oslo, 1955).

17. E. Gurney Clark and Niels Danbolt, "The Oslo Study of the Natural Course of Untreated Syphilis: An Epidemiologic Investigation Based on a Restudy of the Boeck-Bruusgaard Material," *Journal of Chronic Diseases,* 2:311-344, (September 1955); and *Medical Clinics of North America,* 48:613-623, (May 1964).

18. R. A. Vonderlehr, T. Clark, O. C. Wenger, and J. R. Heller, "Untreated Syphilis in the Male Negro," *Journal of Venereal Disease Information,* 17:260-265 (September 1936).

19. J. R. Heller, Jr., and P. T. Bruyere, "Untreated Syphilis in Male Negro: II Mortality During 12 Years of Observation," *Journal of Venereal Disease Information*, 27:34-38 (February 1946).

20. J. J. Peters, J. H. Peers, S. Olansky, J. C. Cutler, and G. A. Gleeson, "Untreated Syphilis in Male Negro: Pathologic Findings in Syphilitic and Non-syphilitic Patients," *Journal of Chronic Diseases*, 1:127-148 (1955).

21. Paul D. Rosahn, *Autopsy Studies in Syphilis*, PHS Publication No. 433, (Washington, D. C., 1960).

22. R. A. Vonderlehr and L. J. Usilton, "The Chance of Acquiring Syphilis and the Frequency of Its Disastrous Outcome," *Journal of Venereal Disease Information*, 19:396 (November 1938).

23. Adapted from Odin W. Anderson, *Syphilis and Society -- Problems of Control in the United States, 1912-1964* (Chicago, 1965), p. 11.

24. Adapted from R. A. Vonderlehr, "Maternal Education, the Root of Congenital Syphilis Problem," as cited in *Journal of Venereal Disease Information*, 20:349 (November 1939).

25. *VD Fact Sheet, 1964*, PHS Publication No. 341 (Atlanta, Georgia), p. 11.

26. Thomas Parran, *Shadow On the Land* (New York: Reynal and Hitchcock, 1937), p. 177.

27. Clark and Danbolt, "The Oslo Study of the Natural Course of Untreated Syphilis," *Medical Clinics of North America*, p. 622.

28. Joseph Earle Moore, *The Modern Treatment of Syphilis*, 2nd ed. (Baltimore, 1941), p. 263.

29. John H. Stokes, Herman Beerman, and Norman R. Ingraham, *Modern Clinical Syphilology*, 3rd ed. (Philadelphia, 1944), p. 30.

30. Adapted from Rosahn, *Autopsy Studies in Syphilis*.

31. *Vital Statistics of the United States, 1955*, vol. I, p. xxv.

32. Moore, *The Modern Treatment of Syphilis*, p. 284.

33. R. H. Kampmeier, "The Late Manifestations of Syphilis: Skeletal, Visceral, and Cardiovascular," *Medical Clinics of North America*, 48:692-699 (May 1964).

34. Rosahn, *Autopsy Studies in Syphilis*, p. 60.

35. Stokes, Beerman, and Ingraham, *Modern Clinical Syphilology*, pp. 904-905.

36. Kampmeier, "The Late Manifestations of Syphilis," p. 690.

37. James F. Donohue and Quentin R. Remein, "Long-Term Trend and Economic Factors of Paresis in the United States," *Public Health Reports*, 69:758-765 (August 1954).

38. Moore, *The Modern Treatment of Syphilis*, p. 366.

39. Benjamin Malzberg, *Cohort Studies of Mental Disease in New York State, 1943-1949* (New York, 1958), p. 30.

40. Morton Kramer, "Long Range Studies of Mental Hospital Patients: An Important Area for Research in Chronic Disease," *The Milbank Memorial Fund Quarterly*, 31:253-264 (July 1953).

41. Donohue and Remein, "Long-Term Trend and Economic Factors of Paresis in the United States."

42. *VD Fact Sheet, 1952*, PHS Publication No. 341, p. 5.

43. *VD Fact Sheet, 1967,* 24th Revision, PHS Publication, p. 4.

44. Evan W. Thomas, "Some Aspects of Neurosyphilis," *Medical Clinics of North America,* 48:699-706 (May 1964).

45. *VD Fact Sheet, 1965,* PHS Publication No. 341, p. 8.

46. Harold A. Kahn and Albert P. Iskrant, "Syphilis Mortality Analysis, 1933-45," *Journal of Venereal Disease Information,* 29:193-200 (July 1948).

47. Edith C. Kerby, "Causes of Blindness in Children of School Age," *The Sight-Saving Review,* 28:10-21 (Spring 1958).

48. Monroe Lerner and Odin W. Anderson, *Health Progress in the United States, 1900-1960* (Chicago, 1963), p. 209.

49. Kerby, "Causes of Blindness in Children of School Age," pp. 10-21.

50. Lerner and Anderson, *Health Progress in the United States, 1900-1960,* p. 209.

51. Louis Dublin, *The Facts of Life* (New York: The Macmillan Co., 1951), p. 335.

52. Thorstein Guthe, "Measure of the Treponematoses Problem in the World," *World Forum On Syphilis and Other Treponematoses,* PHS Publication No. 997 (Washington, D. C., 1964), pp. 11-20.

53. *VD Fact Sheet,* 1967, 24th Revision, PHS Publication, p. 4.

Chapter 8. Venereal Disease in the Military

1. Joseph Siler, "The Prevention and Control of Venereal Diseases in the Army of the United States of America," *Army Medical Bulletin No. 67,* (Pennsylvania, 1943), p. 135.

2. Josephine Hinrichsen, "Venereal Disease in Major Armies and Navies of the World," *American Journal of Syphilis, Gonorrhea, and Venereal Diseases,* 28: 736-772 (November 1944); 29: 80-124 (January 1945); and 29: 229-267 (March 1945).

3. Siler, "The Prevention and Control of Venereal Diseases in the Army of the United States of America," p. 209.

4. John B. Coates, ed., *Preventive Medicine in World War II: Communicable Diseases Transmitted by Contact or by Unknown Means,* vol. V (Washington, D. C., 1960), p. 146.

5. Siler, "The Prevention and Control of Venereal Diseases in the Army of the United States of America."

Chapter 9. International Venereal Disease Control

1. John E. Gordon, ed., *Control of Communicable Diseases in Man,* 10th ed. (New York: American Public Health Association, 1965), p. 266.

2. *Ibid.,* p. 164.

3. *Ibid.,* p. 236.

4. Thorstein Guthe, "Measure of the Treponematoses Problem in the World," *World Forum on Syphilis and Other Treponematoses,* PHS Publication No. 997 (Washington, D. C., 1964), pp. 11-20.

Chapter 10. Chancroid, Lymphogranuloma Venereum, and Granuloma Inguinale

1. Franklin H. Top, ed., *Communicable and Infectious Diseases,* 5th ed. (St. Louis, 1964), p. 612.

2. Ibid., p. 663.

Bibliography

Abraham, J. Johnston. "Some Account of the History of the Treatment of Syphilis," *British Journal of Venereal Diseases*, 24:153-160 (December 1948).

Ackerman, A. B., and R. Calabria. "Asymptomatic Gonorrhea and the Gonococcal Carrier State, and Gonococcemia in Men," *Journal of the American Medical Association*, 196:101-103 (April 4, 1966).

Anderson, Odin W. *Syphilis and Society: Problems of Control in the United States, 1912-1964*. Center for Health Administration Studies, Research Series 22. Chicago: University of Chicago, 1965.

Anderson, Otis L. "The Control of Venereal Diseases Among Industrial Workers," *American Journal of Syphilis, Gonorrhea, and Venereal Diseases*, 27:432-438 (July 1943).

Bauer, Theodore J. "Half a Century of International Control of the Venereal Diseases," *Public Health Reports*, 68:779-787 (August 1953).

Beerman, Herman. "The Problem of Reinoculation of Human Beings with *Spirochaeta Pallida*," *American Journal of Syphilis, Gonorrhea, and Venereal Diseases*, 30:173-192 (March 1946).

Bowdoin, C. D. "Mass Blood Testing in Eight Georgia Communities," *Journal of Venereal Disease Information*, 29:126-131 (May 1948).

Brown, Earle G. "A Study of Venereal Disease Prevalence in 22 Kansas Counties," *Venereal Disease Information*, 9:185-191 (May 1928).

Brown, William J., and J. A. Mahoney. "Serologic Tests for Syphilis: A Profile of Hospital Practice," *Journal of the American Hospital Association*, 37:65-69 (November 1963).

Brown, William J., and E. J. Sunkes. "A Recent Study of Results of Premarital Serologic Testing in a Southern State," *Southern Medical Journal*, 52:707-710 (June 1959).

Brunet, Walter M. "Venereal Disease Prevalence in the City of New York: Kings County (Brooklyn) – II," *Long Island Medical Journal*, 23:158-172 (March 1929).

Brunet, Walter M., and Mary S. Edwards. "A Survey of Venereal Disease Prevalence in Detroit," *Venereal Disease Information*, 8:197-208 (June 1927).

Bruusgaard, Edvin. "Uber das Schicksal der nicht spezifisch behandelten Luetiker," *Archiv fur Dermatologie und Syphilis*, 157:309 (1929).

Clark, E. Gurney, and Niels Danbolt. "The Oslo Study of the Natural History of Untreated Syphilis: An Epidemiologic Investigation Based on a Restudy of the Boeck-Bruusgaard Material," *Journal of Chronic Diseases*, 2:311-344 (September 1955).

––– "The Oslo Study of the Natural History of Untreated Syphilis: An Epidemiologic Investigation Based on a Restudy of the Boeck-Bruusgaard Material," *Medical Clinics of North America*, vol. 48, no. 3 (May 1964), pp. 613-623.

Clark, Taliaferro, and Elizabeth V. Milovich. "Prevalence of Venereal Diseases in Charleston, West Virginia," *Venereal Disease Information*, 12:259-267 (June 1931).

Clark, Taliaferro, and Lida J. Usilton. "Survey of the Venereal Diseases in the City of Baltimore, Baltimore County, and the Four Contiguous Counties," *Venereal Disease Information,* 12:437-456 (October 1931).

Clark, Taliaferro, L. J. Usilton, and F. D. Stricker. "Trend of Venereal Diseases in Oregon," *Northwest Medicine,* 32:265-272 (July 1933).

Coates, John B., ed. *Preventive Medicine in World War II: Communicable Diseases Transmitted by Contact or by Unknown Means,* vol. V. Office of the Surgeon General, Department of the Army. Washington, D.C.: U.S. Government Printing Office, 1960.

Cockburn, Thomas A. *The Evolution and Eradication of Infectious Diseases.* Baltimore: Johns Hopkins Press, 1963.

Cohen, I. R. "Natural and Immune Human Antibodies Reactive with Antigens of Virulent *Neisseria Gonorrhoeae,* Immunoglobulins G, M, and A." In publication.

Cole, Harold N. "Antiquity of Syphilis with Some Observations on Its Treatment Through the Ages," *Archives of Dermatology and Syphilology,* 64:12-22 (July 1951).

"Comparability Ratios Based on Mortality Statistics for the Fifth and Sixth Revisions: United States 1950," *Vital Statistics–Special Reports,* vol. 51, no. 3 (1964), pp. 179-246.

"Comparability of Mortality Statistics for the Sixth and Seventh Revisions: United States, 1958," *Vital Statistics–Special Reports,* vol. 51, no. 4 (1965), pp. 247-297.

Condit, P. K., and A. Frank Brewer. "Premarital Examination Laws–Are They Worthwhile? California Experience with 2,000,000 Examinations," *American Journal of Public Health,* 48:880 (July 1953).

"Control of Gonococcal Infections," *World Health Organization Chronical,* 18:14-15 (January 1964).

Curtis, Arthur C. "National Survey of Venereal Disease Treatment," *Journal of the American Medical Association,* 186:46-49 (October 1963).

Dattner, Bernhard. *The Management of Neurosyphilis.* New York: Grune and Stratton, Inc., 1944.

Davis, David J. "The Medical History of the Four Voyages of Columbus," *Proceedings of the Institute of Medicine of Chicago,* 18:363-365 (October 1951).

Deacon, W. E. "Fluorescent Antibody Methods for *Neisseria Gonorrhoeae* Identification," *World Health Organization Bulletin,* 24:349-355 (1961).

Donohue, James F., and Quentin R. Remein. "Long-Term Trend and Economic Factors of Paresis in the United States," *Public Health Reports,* vol. 69, no. 8 (August 1954), pp. 758-765.

Dublin, Louis I., and Mortimer Spiegelman. *The Facts of Life: From Birth to Death.* New York: The Macmillan Co., 1951.

Dubos, Rene, ed. *Bacterial and Mycotic Infections in Man,* 4th ed. Philadelphia: J. B. Lippincott Co., 1965.

Dunn, Halbert L., and William Shackley. "Comparison of Cause-of-Death Assignments by the 1929 and 1938 Revisions of the International List: Deaths in the United States, 1940," *Vital Statistics–Special Reports,* vol. 19, no. 14 (1944), pp. 153-278.

Eagle, Harry. *The Laboratory Diagnosis of Syphilis.* St. Louis: C. V. Mosby Co., 1937.

——— "On the Specificity of Serologic Tests for Syphilis as Determined by 40,545 Tests in a College Student Population," *American Journal of Syphilis, Gonorrhea, and Venereal Diseases,* 25:7-15 (1941).

Edwards, Mary S. "A Census of Cases of Syphilis and Gonorrhea Under Treatment in Philadelphia," *Venereal Disease Information,* 11:1-12 (January 1930).

The Eradication of Syphilis. A Task Force Report to the Surgeon General Public Health Service on Syphilis Control in the United States. Public Health Service Publication No. 918. Washington, D.C.: U.S. Government Printing Office, 1962.

Findings on the Serologic Test for Syphilis in Adults: United States, 1960-1962. U.S. Department of Health, Education, and Welfare, Public Health Service Publication No. 1000, Series 11, No. 9. Washington, D.C.: U.S. Government Printing Office, 1965.

Fiumara, Nicholas J. "The Diagnosis of Gonorrhea," *Tufts Folia Medica,* 8:121-124 (October-December 1962).

——— "Sic Semper Syphilis," *The Boston Medical Quarterly,* 8:101-109 (December 1957).

Fleming, William L. "Syphilis Through the Ages," *Medical Clinics of North America,* 48:587-612 (May 1964).

Gjestland, Trygve. "The Oslo Study of Untreated Syphilis: An Epidemiologic Investigation of the Natural Course of Untreated Syphilis Based on a Restudy of the Boeck-Bruusgaard Material." *Acta Dermato-Venereologica,* vol. 35, supplementum 34 (Oslo, 1955).

The Gonococcus. Public Health Service Publication No. 499. Washington, D.C.: U.S. Government Printing Office, 1962.

"Gonorrhea, Interim Recommended Treatment Schedules, July 1965." Insert in *Notes on Modern Management of V.D.* Public Health Service Publication No. 859. Washington, D.C.: U.S. Government Printing Office, 1962.

Goodman, Herman. *Notable Contributors to the Knowledge of Syphilis.* New York: Medical Lay Press, 1953.

Gordon, John E., ed. *Control of Communicable Diseases in Man,* 10th ed. New York: American Public Health Association, 1965.

Gray, A. L., Howard Boone, and Richard S. Hibbets. "Venereal Disease Case-finding in Quitman County, Mississippi," *Journal of Venereal Disease Information,* 30:127-130 (May 1949).

Gray, A. L., Mary Sim Ferguson, and Richard S. Hibbets. "Delta Plantation Casefinding Survey in LeFlore County, Mississippi," *Journal of Venereal Disease Information,* 29:106-110 (April 1948).

Greenblatt, Robert B., E. R. Pund, E. S. Sanderson, Richard Torpin, and R. B. Dienst. *Management of Chancroid, Granuloma Inquinale, Lymphogranuloma Venereum in General Practice.* Public Health Service Publication No. 255. Washington, D.C.: U.S. Government Printing Office, 1953.

Guthe, Thorstein. "Measure of the Treponematoses Problem in the World," in *Proceedings of World Forum on Syphilis and Other Treponematoses* (September 4-8, 1962). Public Health Service Publication No. 997. Washington, D.C.: U.S. Government Printing Office, 1964, pp. 11-20.

Harrison, L. W. "The Origin of Syphilis," *British Journal of Venereal Diseases*, 35:1-7 (March 1959).

Heller, J. R., Jr., and P. T. Bruyere. "Untreated Syphilis in Male Negro: II. Mortality During 12 Years of Observation," *Journal of Venereal Disease Information*, 27:34-38 (1946).

Hinrichsen, Josephine. "Venereal Disease in Major Armies and Navies of the World," *American Journal of Syphilis, Gonorrhea, and Venereal Diseases*, 28:736-772 (November 1944); 29:80-124 (January 1945); and 29:229-267 (March 1945).

Holcomb, R. C. "The Antiquity of Congenital Syphilis," *Bulletin of Historical Medicine*, 10:148-177 (1941).

——— "Christopher Columbus and the American Origin of Syphilis," *United States Naval Medical Bulletin*, 32:401-430 (1934).

Hudson, Ellis H. "Treponematosis and African Slavery," *British Journal of Venereal Diseases*, 40:43-52 (March 1964).

——— "Treponematosis and Anthropology," *Annals of Internal Medicine*, 58:1037-48 (June 1963).

——— "Treponematosis and Pilgrimage," *American Journal of the Medical Sciences*, 246:645-656 (December 1963).

Kahn, Harold A., and Albert P. Iskrant. "Syphilis Mortality Analysis 1933-45," *Journal of Venereal Disease Information*, 29:193-200 (July 1948).

Kampmeier, Rudolph H. *Essentials of Syphilology*. Philadelphia: J. B. Lippincott Co., 1944.

——— "The Late Manifestations of Syphilis: Skeletal, Visceral and Cardio-vascular," *Medical Clinics of North America*, 48:667-696 (May 1964).

Kellogg, D. S., Jr., and W. E. Deacon, "A New Rapid Immunofluorescent Staining Technique for Identification of *Treponema pallidum* and *Neisseria Gonorrhoeae*," *Proceedings of the Society for Experimental Biology and Medicine*, 115:963-965 (1964).

Kerby, Edith C. "Causes of Blindness in Children of School Age," *The Sight-Saving Review*, 28:10-21 (1958).

King, Ambrose. *Recent Advances in Venereology*. Boston: Little, Brown and Co., 1964.

Kolmer, John A., and Elsa R. Lynch. "False Positive Reactions in the Serologic Diagnosis of Syphilis," *American Journal of Clinical Pathology*, 23:854-865 (September 1953).

Kramer, Morton. "Long Range Studies of Mental Hospital Patients, An Important Area for Research in Chronic Disease," *The Milbank Memorial Fund Quarterly*, vol. 31, no. 3 (July 1953), pp. 36-46.

Lentz, John W., and Herman Beerman. "The Treatment of Venereal Diseases in Private Practice in Philadelphia," *American Journal of Syphilis, Gonorrhea, and Venereal Diseases*, 37:427-438 (September 1953).

Lerner, Monroe, and Odin W. Anderson. *Health Progress in the United States, 1900-1960*. Chicago: University of Chicago Press, 1963.

Magnuson, Harold J., Evan W. Thomas, Sidney Olansky, Bernard I. Kaplan, Lopo De Mello, and John C. Cutler. "Inoculation Syphilis in Human Volunteers," *Medicine*, 35:33-82 (February 1956).

Magnusson, B., and J. Kjellander, "Gonococcal Complement-fixation Test in Complicated and Uncomplicated Gonorrhea," *British Journal of Venereal Diseases,* 41:127-131 (June 1965).

Mahoney, J. F., et al. "Experimental Gonococcic Urethritis in Human Volunteers," *American Journal of Syphilis, Gonorrhea, and the Venereal Diseases,* 30:1 (January 1946).

Mahoney, J. F., R. D. Arnold, and A. Harris. "Penicillin Treatment of Early Syphilis: A Preliminary Report," *Journal of Venereal Disease Information,* 24:355-357 (December 1943).

Malzberg, Benjamin. *Cohort Studies of Mental Disease in New York State, 1943-1949.* New York: National Association for Mental Health, 1958.

Mann, Charles H. "Seventy-five Years of Progress in Venereal Disease Therapy," *Quarterly Review of Internal Medicine and Dermatology,* 8:264-266 (December 1951).

Martin, J. E., W. L. Peacock, and J. D. Thayer. "Further Studies with a Selective Medium for Cultivating *Neisseria Gonorrhoeae*," *British Journal of Venereal Diseases,* 41:199-201 (September 1965).

Medical News Section, *Journal of the American Medical Association,* 193:23-24 (August 23, 1965).

Miller, P. C., M. J. Drell, V. Moeller, and M. Bohnhoff. "Experimental Gonococcal Infection of the Rabbit's Eye," *Journal of Infectious Diseases,* 77:193-200 (1945).

Miller, P. C. "Experimental Gonococcal Infection," in *Gonococcus and Gonococcal Infection.* The American Association for the Advancement of Science, Publication No. 11. Lancaster, Pa.: The Science Press, 1939, pp. 20-22.

Miller, Seward E. *A Textbook of Clinical Pathology.* Baltimore: The Williams and Wilkins Co., 1955.

Milovich, Elizabeth V. "A Study of Venereal Disease Prevalence in Mississippi," *Venereal Disease Information,* 10:208:224 (May 1929).

Moore, George, and Malcolm T. Foster. "Selective Casefinding in Syphilis Control," *Public Health Reports,* 68:167-172 (February 1953).

Moore, Joseph Earle. *The Modern Treatment of Syphilis,* 2nd ed. Baltimore: Charles C. Thomas, 1941.

Moore, Joseph Earle, and Charles F. Mohr. "Biologically False Positive Serologic Tests for Syphilis," *Journal of the American Medical Association,* 150:467-473 (October 1952).

Moore, M. Brittain, Eleanor V. Price, John M. Knox, and Lee W. Elgin. "Epidemiologic Treatment of Contacts to Infectious Syphilis," *Public Health Reports,* 78:966-970 (November 1963).

Morse, John W., and A. P. Iskrant. "Syphilis Casefinding Through Education," *Journal of Venereal Disease Information,* 32:150-157 (June 1951).

A National Study of Venereal Disease Incidence: Summary Report. New York: American Social Health Association, 1963.

"New Edition of Hospital Accreditation Standards," *Journal of the American Medical Association,* 161:242 (May 1956).

Nicoll, M., and M. T. Bellows. "Effect of a Confidential Inquiry on the Recorded Mortality from Syphilis and Alcoholism," *American Journal of Public Health,* 24:813-820 (1934).

Pariser, H., A. D. Farmer, and A. F. Marino. "Asymptomatic Gonorrhea in the Male," *Southern Medical Journal*, 57:680-690 (June 1964).

Parran, Thomas. "Are We Stamping Out Syphilis?" as cited in Odin W. Anderson, *Syphilis and Society*. Center for Health Administration Studies, Research Series 22. Chicago: University of Chicago, 1965.

————*Shadow On the Land*. New York: Reynal & Hitchcock, 1937.

Parran, Thomas, et al. "Venereal Disease Prevalence in Cleveland," *Bulletin of the Academy of Medicine of Cleveland*, 12:5-10, 19 (August 1928).

Parran, Thomas, Willard C. Smith, and Selwyn D. Collins. "Venereal Disease Prevalence in 14 Communities," *Venereal Disease Information*, 9:45-60 (February 1928).

Peacock, W. L., Jr., and J. D. Thayer. "Direct Fluorescent Antibody Technique Using Flazo Orange Counterstain in Identification of *Neisseria Gonorrhoeae*," *Public Health Reports*, 79:1119-22 (December 1964).

Pelouze, Percy P. *Gonorrhea in the Male and Female*. Philadelphia: W. B. Saunders Co., 1941.

Peters, J. J., J. H. Peers, S. Olansky, J. C. Cutler, and G. A. Gleeson. "Untreated Syphilis in Male Negro: Pathologic Findings in Syphilitic and Nonsyphilitic Patients," *Journal of Chronic Diseases*, 1:127-148 (February 1955).

Pfeiffer, Albert, and Herbert W. Cummings. "A One-Day Incidence Study of Syphilis and Gonorrhea in New York State," *Venereal Disease Information*, 9:143-151 (April 1928).

Pohlen, Kurt. "The Frequency of Syphilis and Its Sequels According to Clinical and Autopsy Findings." *Dermatologische Wochenschrift*, 105:1469 (Leipzig, November 1937), as abstracted in *Journal of Venereal Disease Information*, vol. 19, no. 6 (June 1938), p. 184.

Proceedings of the World Forum on Syphilis and Other Treponematoses. Public Health Service Publication No. 997. Washington, D.C.: U.S. Government Printing Office, 1964.

Pusey, William A. *The History and Epidemiology of Syphilis*. Springfield, Ill.: Charles C. Thomas, 1933.

Reising, G., and D. S. Kellogg, Jr., "Detection of Gonococcal Antibody," *Proceedings of Society Experimental, Biology, and Medicine*, 120:660-663 (1965).

Rockwell, Donald H., Anne R. Yobs, and M. Brittain Moore. "The Tuskegee Study of Untreated Syphilis," *Archives of Internal Medicine*, 114:792-798 (December 1964).

Rosahn, P. D. *Autopsy Studies in Syphilis*. Public Health Service Publication No. 433. Washington, D.C.: U.S. Government Printing Office, 1960.

Schamberg, Ira L., and Howard P. Steiger. "Syphilitic Relapse vs. Reinfection," *Journal of Venereal Disease Information*, 29:92-103 (April 1948).

Serologic Tests for Syphilis. Public Health Service Publication No. 411. Washington, D.C.: U.S. Government Printing Office, 1964.

Siler, Joseph F. "The Prevention and Control of Venereal Diseases in the Army of the United States of America," *Army Medical Bulletin* No. 67. Special Issue Pennsylvania: Carlisle Barracks, May 1943.

Smith, W. H. Y., Lida J. Usilton, and Martha C. Bruyere. "Syphilis Control Through Mass Blood Testing," *Venereal Disease Information,* 26:130-133 (June 1945).

Smith, Willard C. "Venereal Disease Prevalence in St. Louis," *Venereal Disease Information,* 10:189-208 (May 1929).

Sparling P. F., A. R. Yobs, T. E. Billings, and J. F. Hackney. "Spectinomycin Sulfate and Aqueous Procaine Penicillin G. in Treatment of Female Gonorrhea Antimicrobial Agents and Chemotherapy—1965," *Antimicrobial Agents and Chemotherapy* (American Society for Microbiology, 1965), 5:689-692.

Stokes, John H. *Modern Clinical Syphilology,* 2nd ed. Philadelphia: W. B. Saunders Co., 1934.

Stokes, John H., Herman Beerman, and Norman R. Ingraham, Jr. *Modern Clinical Syphilology,* 3rd ed. Philadelphia: W. B. Saunders Co., 1944.

Stokes, John H., Herman Beerman, and Norman R. Ingraham. "Syphilis in Industry: A Review of Problems and Policy," *American Journal of the Medical Sciences,* 196:600-608 (October 1938).

Syphilis Epidemiology, Report No. 2, U.S. Department of Health, Education and Welfare, Public Health Service, Communicable Disease Center (Atlanta, Georgia, July 23, 1965), p. 14.

Syphilis: Modern Diagnosis and Management. Public Health Service Publication No. 743. Washington, D.C.: U.S. Government Printing Office, 1961.

Taggert, Ross, T. Morgan, and J. Tendleton. "District of Columbia Blood Testing Survey for Syphilis in Selected Industries and Trades," *Medical Annals of the District of Columbia,* 25:73-76 (February 1956).

Thayer, James D., and J. E. Martin, Jr., "A Selective Medium for the Cultivation of *Neisseria Gonorrhoeae* and *Neisseria Meningitidis,*" *Public Health Reports,* 79:49-57 (January 1964).

——— "Improved Medium Selective for Cultivation of *Neisseria Gonorrhoeae* and *Neisseria Meningitidis,*" *Public Health Reports,* 81:559-562 (June 1966).

Thayer, James D., and M. B. Moore, Jr. "Gonorrhea—Present Knowledge, Research, and Control Efforts," *Medical Clinics of North America,* 48:762 (May 1964).

Thomas, Evan W. "Some Aspects of Neurosyphilis," *Medical Clinics of North America,* 48:699-706 (May 1964).

———*Syphilis: Its Course and Management.* New York: The Macmillan Co., 1949.

Today's VD Control Problem: Joint Statement. Association of State and Territorial Health Officers, American Venereal Disease Association, and American Social Health Association. New York, March 1964.

Today's VD Control Problem: Joint Statement. The American Public Health Association, The American Social Health Association, The American Venereal Disease Association, The Association of State and Territorial Health Officers with the cooperation of the American Medical Association. New York, January 1967.

Today's VD Control Problem: Joint Statement. Association of State and Territorial Health Officers, American Venereal Disease Association, and American Social Health Association, New York, March 1965.

Top, Franklin H., ed. *Communicable and Infectious Diseases*, 5th ed. St. Louis: C. V. Mosby Co., 1964.

Trythall, S. W. "The Premarital Law: History and Survey in Michigan," *Journal of the American Medical Association*, 187:900 (June 1964).

Usilton, Lida J. "Venereal Disease Prevalence in Tennessee," *Venereal Disease Information*, 9:419-443 (October 1928).

Usilton, Lida J., and W. D. Riley. "Venereal Disease Prevalence in Virginia," *Virginia Medical Monthly*, 57:389-397 (September 1930).

Van Buren, George H. "Some Things You Can't Prove by Mortality Statistics," *Vital Statistics—Special Reports*, vol. 12, no. 13, p. 191-209, 1940.

VD Fact Sheet. Public Health Service Publication No. 341. U. S. Department of Health, Education, and Welfare, Public Health Service, Communicable Disease Center, Atlanta, Georgia. Published annually 1947–1965.

Venereal Disease Branch Report, Fiscal Year 1966. U. S. Department of Health, Education, and Welfare, Public Health Service, Communicable Disease Center, Venereal Disease Branch, Atlanta, Georgia, 1966.

Venereal Disease in Canada, Annual Report, 1964. Epidemiology Division, Department of National Health and Welfare, Ottawa, Canada.

Vital Statistics Rates in the United States, 1900-1940. Vital Statistics Division, National Center for Health Statistics. Washington, D.C.: U.S. Government Printing Office, 1943.

Vital Statistics of the United States, published annually, 1900 to date. Vital Statistics Division, National Center for Health Statistics. Washington, D.C.: U.S. Government Printing Office.

Vonderlehr, R. A. "Maternal Education the Root of the Congenital Syphilis Problem," *Health Officer* 4:118 (July-August 1939), as cited in *Journal of Venereal Disease Information*, 20:349 (November 1939).

Vonderlehr, R. A., and L. J. Usilton. "The Chance of Acquiring Syphilis and the Frequency of Its Disastrous Outcome," *Journal of Venereal Disease Information*, 19:396 (November 1938).

Vonderlehr, R. A., T. Clark, O. C. Wenger, and J. R. Heller. "Untreated Syphilis in Male Negro." *Journal of Venereal Disease Information*, 17:260-265 (1936).

White, L. A., and D. S. Kellogg, Jr., *"Neisseria Gonorrhoeae* Identification in Direct Smears by a Fluorescent Antibody-Counterstain Method," *Applied Microbiology*, 13:171-173 (March 1965).

White, Paul C., and Joseph H. Blount. "Venereal Disease Control in the 2nd Marine Division, Camp Lejeune, North Carolina," *Military Medicine*, 132:252-257 (April 1967).

Wilcox, R. R. "Venereal Disease in the Bible," *British Journal of Venereal Diseases*, 25:28-33 (March 1949).

Wilkinson, A. E., "A Note on the Use of Thayer and Martin's Selective Medium for *Neisseria Gonorrhoeae*," *British Journal of Venereal Diseases*, 4:60-61 (March 1965).

Williams Herbert U. "The Origin and Antiquity of Syphilis: The Evidence of Diseased Bones," *Archives of Pathology*, 13:931-983 (June 1932).

Index